Happiness Triggers

The Science of Moving from
Happiness to Empowered Joy

Second Edition

By
Christian Frazier

Foreword By

Joe Bohn, PhD, MBA

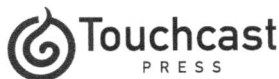

Touchcast
PRESS

Dedication

To all of those who have experienced trauma, pain, setbacks, and challenges this book is dedicated to you. It is for every person who has felt broken, unseen, or stuck in cycles of suffering, yet still carried within them the hope of something more. You are the heartbeat of these pages.

When I first released *Happiness Triggers*, I could not have imagined the overwhelming response. The reviews came pouring in: readers called it ***"life-changing"* and *"a must-read."*** Counselors and coaches praised it as an evidence-based, science-backed guide that speaks to both the heart and the mind. Fathers and sons told me they were reading it together and finding healing conversations they never thought possible. Families shared that it was reshaping how they communicated at the dinner table. Some described it as "therapy in book form," others as a mirror that reflected their pain back to them but with a light of hope they hadn't seen in years. The response was far greater than anything I expected, and the fact that a university has chosen to include *Happiness Triggers* in its syllabus is proof that its impact is not only personal but generational.

And then life tested me. Not long after writing this book, a hurricane ripped the roof off my home, leaving me unhoused and living in a hotel for five months. Just as I finally settled into a new place, I received sobering health news: I was at high risk for a stroke or aneurysm. For months I lived with the weight of uncertainty, believing an incident could strike at any moment. I eventually underwent a brain procedure that revealed everything was okay, but those months forced me to practice what I preach. I leaned into mindfulness, self-care, and gratitude. I refused to let fear silence me. I committed to *thinking from the finish line* to seeing myself healed and whole, even in the face of uncertainty. It doesn't mean that I didn't have fear but I had the power to press through my fears.

Through it all, I still showed up for others. I still taught. I still served, I still inspired, and I learned firsthand that *my purpose doesn't pause for pain*. That truth deepened not just my life, but this book.

Out of these experiences grew new programs: *Happiness Triggers in the Workplace* and *Happiness Triggers in Higher Education*. From corporate boardrooms to college classrooms, the tools in this book are helping people break free from burnout, build resilience, and reclaim joy in environments that need it most.

This **second edition** is more than a continuation, it is a testimony. *Happiness Triggers* is no longer just my story; it belongs to all of us. It is a reminder that no matter the storm, no matter the diagnosis, no matter the pain, joy can still be rebuilt, reclaimed, and lived out loud.

Praise for Happiness Triggers

"When I first started reading *Happiness Triggers*, I recognized the essence of it immediately. This book identifies how individuals have used the identified proven psychological principles to control irrational thoughts and reduce unwanted negative behaviors. There are easy to understand explanations and examples of individual changes using these psychological principles to improve daily functioning and happiness. In fact, they are the same therapeutic principles and goals that I have used with my clients in private practice as a licensed psychotherapist."

Tommy Childers, PhD
Licensed Mental Health Counselor
Certified Clinical Mental Health Counselor
National Certified Counselor

***

"Our mental health and wholeness is a precious gift to be cherished. Many people struggle unnecessarily not knowing a song would lift them or a self-affirmation would uncap the well of hidden joy. This book is the "been there, done that," t-shirt for the masses. Dr. Frazier passionately offers this start to mental health and wholeness. Singing, affirming, letting it go and more are the Happiness Triggers so desperately needed today."

Rev. Dr. Alec D. Richardson - Founding Pastor of Greater
Dimensions Christian
Assembly

iv

***

"In Happiness Triggers, Rev. Dr. Christian Frazier offers a profound and practical guide to mental well-being, rooted in his own transformative journey and learned experiences from others; a testimony to the fact, that Happiness is a State of Mind, which I learned as a child.

This book goes beyond simple advice, while providing a toolkit for resilience, mindfulness, and intentional living. Dr. Frazier's ability to blend personal experience with actionable strategies creates a resource that is both accessible and deeply insightful. Through each chapter, he invites us to not only reconsider our approach to happiness, but to actively shape it—empowering us to reclaim joy, even in life's most challenging moments; thus reminding us that happiness is indeed a State of Mind and practicable."

Rasul Ramji, DC, DrPH
Author of *Once Upon a Dream. A Tale of Fated Love*

***

"Happiness Triggers has something for every reader of this book that will give you a fresh wind in your life accompanied by resilience and the tenacity to win. Through my own personal journey of Adverse Childhood Experience after the loss of my mother who died by suicide in my youth, the ability to bounce back from my own struggle from this tragedy inspired me to become a mental health advocate like Christian."

Dr. Terence O. Hayes, Sr.
Board Certified Mental Health Coach
Senior Pastor: Faith Deliverance Church of God in Christ
www.faithdeliverancecogic.net
https://bold.org/donor/drterence-o-hayes-sr/

***

"Happiness Triggers equips individuals to navigate life's challenges while fostering resilience and a renewed sense of purpose. Dr. Frazier's ability to connect timeless evidence-based truths with modern living makes this work a practical guide and essential for anyone seeking to experience happiness. Whether you're an educator, or simply on a journey of self-discovery, Happiness Triggers is an inspiration to embrace joy and purpose. This book is a beacon of hope for our times, and I highly recommend it to readers everywhere."

Dr. Emery Ailes
President, LIFELINE University

***

"Dr. Christian Frazier's Happiness Triggers is engaging, educational, contemplative, and actionable. The design of this book beautifully blends academia with resources listed for further exploration, humor and candor that normalizes the human experience, and gentle invitations for personal growth germane to a mindset of happiness and, ultimately, freedom.

Dr. Frazier shares merited life lessons while daring to be vulnerable and it pays off as the content fosters a keenly felt sense of kindred wisdom."

Amanda Marker, LMHC
Director of Business Development, Windmoor Healthcare
of Clearwater

***

"Dr Frazier's ideas and messages in Happiness Triggers were an awakening in our lives. Whether it is dealing with family matters, work life or health issues, this book will help you recognize how to leverage happiness triggers in for better mental health. His second edition has two new chapters. The chapter on domestic violence a is a must read for everyone to help us quit making excuses for the violence and to make a plan for action. The chapter on happiness trigger ideas for our nation's veterans and first responders gives even more importance to support them as they strengthen hope and make our nation a safer place."

Kristi Franz
Medical Assistant - Clark County School System

Vicki Bohn
Realtor/Broker w/ Semonin Realtors

"Here, Dr. Frazier shares his own life experiences and hard-won insights, making the book feel like a more personal one-on-one conversation with each of his readers."

Rev. J.M. Wiser

About the Author

Rev. Dr. Christian Frazier, CEO of Elevated Minds Coaching, is a highly sought-after corporate wellness consultant, speaker, and workshop facilitator represented by All American Speakers Bureau. As a Certified Life Coach, Nationally Certified Mental Health First Aid Instructor, Health & Nutrition Coach, and Mindfulness Expert, he specializes in helping organizations and individuals achieve success across the eight dimensions of wellness through executive coaching, wellness assessments, and transformative mentoring programs.

A Desert Storm/Desert Shield Gulf War Navy Veteran, Rev. Dr. Frazier brings a unique blend of military discipline, lived experience, and public health approaches to his work. He is nationally recognized for his efforts in raising mental health awareness and reducing suicide rates, utilizing innovative public health strategies in collaboration with the Zero Suicide Alliance and other mental health initiatives. He is a certified Mental Health First Aid instructor and serves as the Chair of the BIPOC Subcommittee and Co-Chair of the Veterans Subcommittee for the Hillsborough Zero Suicide Alliance.

A prolific author, mindfulness expert, and trauma education speaker, Rev. Dr. Frazier has written eight influential books, including *Unleashing Potential* and *Happiness Triggers*, aimed at helping individuals unlock their true potential and live a fulfilled life. As a board member of NAMI Hillsborough and a leader in the National Changing Minds Now Initiative, he continues to champion mental health awareness on both a local and national scale.

Rev. Dr. Christian Frazier is a dynamic advocate, speaker, and thought leader whose work spans multiple industries, from mental health advocacy to media and entertainment. With over 20 years of experience in the field of mental health, Rev. Dr. Frazier is best known for confronting critical societal issues like the Black suicide epidemic and promoting mental wellness, particularly among marginalized communities. His recent features in publications like Parlé Magazine, Bold Journey, and Shoutout Atlanta highlight his tireless efforts to combat the stigma surrounding mental health and encourage open conversations about emotional wellness.

As a media personality, Rev. Dr. Frazier has appeared in numerous articles and television segments, with recognition from major outlets such as The New York Post, The New York Times, and USA Today. He has been honored with prestigious accolades, including being named to the 40 Under 40 and receiving the BE Modern Man award for his impactful work in the community.

Beyond his work in mental health, Rev. Dr. Frazier is a passionate advocate for diabetes awareness and healthy living. As someone who has personally transformed his own health, he shares his journey to inspire others to take control of their wellbeing. His advocacy for healthy lifestyles has earned him recognition across various platforms, including feature articles that discuss his contributions to promoting balanced nutrition, fitness, and mental health as interconnected aspects of overall wellness.

With over two decades as an ordained minister and a Doctor of Ministry, Rev. Dr. Christian Frazier is deeply committed to service. His passion for empowering others through mental health advocacy, personal development, and corporate wellness solutions has made him a standout leader in his field.

In addition to his advocacy, Rev. Dr. Frazier's career in entertainment continues to thrive. From his work as an actor to his roles behind the scenes, his diverse experiences enable him to connect with audiences across all demographics. With a unique blend of charisma, compassion, and expertise, he remains a sought-after speaker, consultant, and mental health educator, bringing hope and resources to those in need.

Parlé Magazine article: <u>Rev. Dr. Christian Frazier Confronts the Black Suicide Epidemic</u>

Bold Journey feature: <u>Meet Christian Frazier - Mental Health Advocate</u>

Shoutout Atlanta interview: <u>Meet Christian Frazier - Mental Health Advocate</u>

ShareCare.com <u>Meet Christian Frazier - Diabetes</u>

PUBLISHED BY
Touchcast Press
Tampa, FL
www.touchcastpress.com
Email: jb@touchcastpress.com

Book cover design by Christian Frazier
Edited by Touchcast Press
Interior design by Touchcast Press

October 2025

Library of Congress Cataloging-in-Publication Data
Library of Congress Control Number: 2025946779

Frazier, Christian
Happiness Triggers. The Science of Moving from Happiness to Empowered Joy. Second Edition / Frazier, Christian—
p. cm.

ISBN: 978-1-966181-06-4 (paperback)
ISBN: 978-1-966181-07-1 (hardcover)
ISBN: 978-1-966181-08-8 (eBook)

1. Happiness. 2. Authenticity. 3. Mental health. 4. Self-care. 5. Self-discovery. 6. Domestic violence. 7. Veterans 8. First responders
I. Title

xi

FOREWORD

For Happiness Triggers, Second Edition

By

Joe Bohn, PhD, MBA

*Life's most persistent and urgent question is,
'What are you doing for others?*

Martin Luther King, Jr.

Mental health, resilience, happiness, mindfulness, authenticity, solitude, and knowing your inner child—all are key concepts and points of discussion throughout this book by Rev. Dr. Christian Frazier. This second edition to his original work, *Happiness Trigger, The Science of Moving from Happiness to Empowered Joy*, Rev. Dr. Frazier has expanded on his practical and common-sense tips and steps for helping all of us live happier and healthier lives.

Three years ago, while working on veteran's suicide prevention outreach community engagement efforts I got introduced to Rev. Dr. Frazier and witnessed his life focus on mental health and wellness advocacy. But he is more than an advocate—he practices what he preaches. Having gone through a series of his own trials, tribulations and transformations in life, he learned many valuable lessons that he has shared with others and has contributed in compiling this book. Anecdotally, when my own sister heard the title of this book she bought a copy. The topics covered and the motivational messages had a profound and positive impact on her along with myself.

Happiness Triggers is based on his experiences working with others and in communities along with key references and his own personalized set of illustrations.

For myself, as with many of us, life has also had its trials and tribulations. As I read over this work by Rev. Dr. Frazier, many of the points he makes resonated including the point that we can all have different happiness triggers starting in Chapter 1. What works for one person may not be applicable for someone else.

This book offers a plethora of ideas to help all of us, regardless of our walk in life or the path that we are traveling. Also, for use as a reading material in colleges and universities, the "Reflective Exercises" and "Journaling Prompts" can aid any instructor with ready-made discussion topics for use in a course.

In this second edition several chapters are updated with new content and illustrations along with a revised Dedication and two new chapters on Happiness Trigger ideas for dealing with domestic violence and for veterans and first responders.

Last, I started this Foreword with a quote from Dr. Martin Luther King, Jr. Dr. King asks us the simple question, "What are you doing for others?" Rev. Dr. Frazier's work embodies a focus on helping others. Since the publishing of his original work, he has shared his Happiness Triggers concepts with others in classes, group meetings, workshops and podcasts. His own work embodies that of this calling from Dr. King, Jr.

Welcome to Rev. Dr. Frazier's journey. It is inspiring, practical and innovative giving each of us something to put into practice in our own journey.

Joe Bohn, PhD, MBA
CEO
Touchcast Press

Happiness Triggers

Table of Contents

Preface

Over the course of my journey—from the military, to the corporate world, and now as a mindfulness and mental health advocate—I have learned that happiness is not a one-size-fits-all concept. It's a deeply personal experience, unique to each individual. However, there are triggers, universal principles, and practices that, when applied consistently, can unlock a sense of joy, resilience, and well-being within all of us. These are what I call "Happiness Triggers," and they are the foundation of this book.

Purpose of This Book

As someone who has navigated the turbulent waters of life—whether through managing talent in the entertainment industry or working directly in mental health advocacy—I've experienced firsthand how critical it is to maintain mental well-being. This book is a reflection of the practices that have helped me reinvent myself time and time again. It's about more than just finding joy—it's about transcending trauma, building resilience, and creating a life anchored in mindfulness and positive action.

Happiness Triggers wasn't an overnight idea—it was born out of years of personal pain, deep research, and dedicated education. It took five years of development before I began sharing the concept, and seeing how it resonated with people confirmed its power to

1

transform lives. The seed was planted in the late 90's at a Tony Robbins event.

When I first began conducting workshops on these principles, I wasn't sure what the response would be. Would people find value in these Happiness Triggers? Would they be able to apply them to their own lives? The feedback I received, however, was overwhelming. Colleagues approached me after workshops with stories of how they planned to implement these triggers in their personal and professional lives. Knowing that these tools are helping others create more joyful and meaningful lives gives me a sense of unspeakable joy. It reinforces my belief that this book is not just an offering of knowledge but a necessary tool to help people transcend their trauma and embrace their full potential.

The artwork featured in *Happiness Triggers Second Edition* was created using artificial intelligence (AI) tools. While the images have been designed to complement the themes and messages within, they are the product of AI's creative capabilities, curated and guided by myself. We acknowledge the role of technology in expanding the boundaries of artistic expression, while ensuring all images serve to enhance the reader's experience.

Intended Audience

The intended audience for *Happiness Triggers* is broad, encompassing anyone looking to unlock greater joy, fulfillment, and emotional well-being in their daily lives. This book is particularly valuable for individuals who have experienced adversity, trauma, or those who are navigating difficult emotional landscapes. Whether you are a professional dealing with workplace stress, a person seeking healing from personal loss or mental health challenges, or someone simply looking to improve your overall happiness, this book offers practical tools and insights that are both empowering and accessible.

By focusing on actionable steps like mindfulness, self-care, and emotional resilience, *Happiness Triggers* equips readers with the tools to reclaim their joy and build lasting emotional strength. The book resonates with those who seek to break free from passive forms of happiness and actively cultivate a life of empowered joy. It's a resource for anyone ready to explore new pathways to mental well-being and create a life that aligns with their deepest values and desires.

Happiness isn't just a feeling that happens to us; it's something we cultivate through mindful choices, resilience, and intention. Through the principles in *Happiness Triggers*, I hope to guide you on your journey toward finding joy, overcoming obstacles, and, ultimately, thriving in every aspect of your life. Together, we will uncover the keys to lasting happiness, anchored in mindfulness and positive psychology.

Thank you for joining me on this transformative journey. May this book be a tool you return to, not just in moments of difficulty, but as a guide to creating a happier, healthier life—one trigger at a time.

With gratitude,

Rev. Dr. Christian Frazier

Chapter 1. Happiness Triggers- A Simple Path to Joy

Starting the Journey

It wasn't until I started working in mental health that I realized something big: growing up poor is a kind of trauma. I had never thought of it that way before. I began hearing words like transgenerational trauma, the idea that fear and pain can be passed down through families, almost like we inherit it in our DNA. Imagine being afraid of things you've never even experienced. That's how deep trauma runs.

I wish I had known about therapy and emotional intelligence back when I was in elementary and middle school. At just seven years old, I was robbed at knife point. Having your life threatened at such a young age is terrifying, but where I grew up, we treated it like "just another day." We normalized it because it was happening to everyone where I grew up in Newark, NJ. Those kinds of experiences aren't normal, they change you. Living in a city where you always have to stay alert, always waiting for someone to try and con you or hurt you, puts your body in constant fight-or-flight mode. Staying on edge like that for years? It changes the chemistry of your brain. It changes the way you think, feel, and see the world.

I was a little odd growing up, different from other kids. What I didn't realize back then was that I was actually gifted. While other kids were out playing, I was reading the dictionary and working my way through an entire set of red encyclopedias my mom bought me. In class, I was always the first one done with assignments, and because I didn't need to study much for tests, I ended up in the back of the room cracking jokes. (They were good ones, too!) My classmates even wrote in my yearbook that I was destined to be a comedian, and funny enough, I actually did become one.

But comedy was just one path. Over time, I studied seminary, computer networking, engineering, human resources, marketing, psychology, and real estate. People used to joke, "What can't you do?" Back then I thought it was all about intelligence. Later I realized it wasn't just being smart, it was believing I could do something, and then taking the steps to actually learn it. There was old school programming language and terms like, "You can't teach an old dog new tricks." Science used to think by the time you were a certain age that we couldn't learn anymore but neuroplasticity tells us that our brains can learn until we leave here.

The truth is, we all have special gifts. Every single one of us. But many of us have been programmed to believe we're limited, to wear masks the world gives us: the mask of our job, our title, our money, our possessions. When you take all of that off, who are you at your core?

That's what this journey through Happiness Triggers is about, learning to peel back the layers, discover your true self, and find out just how much more there is inside you than you ever imagined.

Being You

We all wear masks, our jobs, our titles, our money, our possessions. But when you take all that away, the real question is: Who are you at your core? "Happiness Triggers" will help you discover the answer.

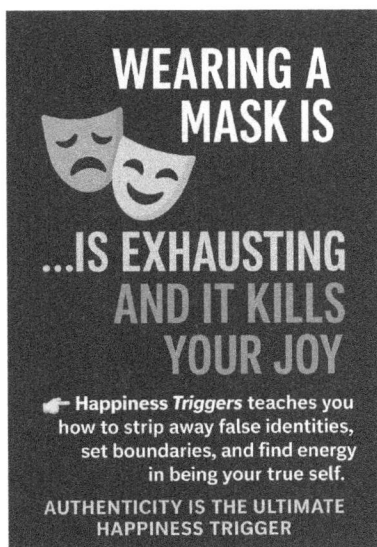

WEARING A MASK IS

...IS EXHAUSTING AND IT KILLS YOUR JOY

Happiness *Triggers* teaches you how to strip away false identities, set boundaries, and find energy in being your true self.

AUTHENTICITY IS THE ULTIMATE HAPPINESS TRIGGER

Let's face it—life can be tough. We're all juggling work, bills, relationships, and countless responsibilities. But somewhere between all the seriousness, we often forget one crucial thing: life is supposed to be fun, too. Remember those childhood days when you could laugh until your belly hurt or play for hours without a care in the world? That carefree joy gets buried as we grow older.

7

Well, here's some good news: it's time to bring that joy back. You don't have to wait for happiness to show up randomly; you can create it.

I've been through my share of challenges—managing talent, producing films, advocating for mental health, you name it. I've also had some hilarious moments, like dealing with diabetes during, uh, less than convenient times. Take that one time my blood sugar dropped during a romantic evening. Let me tell you, nothing throws a wrench in the mood like trying to stay conscious while still...attempting to "raise Lazarus." It's moments like that when you realize life is full of chaos and awkwardness, but also humor if you're willing to see it.

Happiness doesn't come from everything going perfectly. It comes from knowing where to look, what to focus on, and what actions to take. That's where Happiness Triggers come into play.

What Are Happiness Triggers?

Happiness Triggers are simple, intentional actions, thoughts, or habits that can instantly lift your mood. Think of them like buttons you can press when you need to feel better. These triggers won't solve every problem in your life, but they can help you bounce back from stressful moments and create more joy in your everyday routine.

Instead of waiting for happiness to hit you out of no-where, you can trigger it yourself, right when you need it most.

Those Annoying Voices in Your Head

Let's address the elephant in the room—the inner critic. You know, that voice that says things like, "You're not good enough," or "You're going to fail." That voice? It's annoying. And you know what's even more annoying? Those voices usually aren't even ours. They've been planted by other people—teachers, bosses, exes, or even well-meaning family members.

Here's my advice: give those voices names. Not just any name, but the names of people who annoyed you in the past. Maybe it's an old boss, a difficult teacher, or that one "friend" who loved pointing out your flaws. Every time one of those voices comes up, tell them, "Shut up, [insert name here]." It works. You're not just shutting down the negative voices; you're taking back control from whoever first made you doubt yourself.

And when those voices say, "You're not enough," hit back with, "Not only am I enough, I'm more than enough. Where's your proof, huh?" Treat it like an investigative reporter, challenging those baseless claims. Sometimes, it's okay to throw in a few choice words too. Before you know it, that voice will quiet down and start to fall in line.

The Birth of Happiness Triggers

I first got the idea for Happiness Triggers during a Tony Robbins event. Picture this: we were walking across hot coals. Now, the real lesson wasn't just about walking on fire; it was about learning how to shift your emotional state on command. Tony calls it reaching your "peak state," which is all about flipping the switch from fear or stress to confidence and joy in an instant.

That was a turning point for me. If I could learn to manage my emotions in such extreme situations, why not apply the same technique to everyday life? Whether it's a stressful meeting, a tough conversation, or just a bad day, we can use these simple Happiness Triggers to regain control.

The Power of Happiness Triggers

You've probably heard about triggers in the context of trauma—how certain sounds or smells can bring back painful memories. But why not flip the script? Positive triggers can work the same way, but instead of pulling you into negativity, they bring you joy, peace, and energy. And the best part is, you can design your own triggers to fit your unique needs.

The Science Behind Happiness Triggers

Now, I know what you're thinking: "This sounds good, but does it really work?" The answer is yes—and there's science to back it up.

Our brains are wired for something called neuroplasticity, which means they can change and adapt based on our behaviors and thoughts. When you repeatedly focus on positive actions like laughter, mindfulness, or gratitude, your brain literally rewires itself to feel happier.

A 2014 study published in *Social Cognitive and Affective Neuroscience* showed that using positive affirmations can activate the brain's reward centers, making you more resilient to stress.(Cascio, et al., 2014) According to a 2013 Journal of the American Medical Association (*JAMA*) article, mindfulness meditation was shown to be as effective as medication in reducing symptoms of generalized anxiety disorder.(Hoge et al., 2013, p. 174) This means that building Happiness Triggers into your day isn't just a feelgood exercise; it's scientifically proven to boost your mental health. Mindfulness-based stress reduction has been shown to significantly improve mental and physical well-being.(Grossman et al., 2004, p. 38)

Introduction to the Wheel

Happiness is not one thing we chase; it's a balance we create. Imagine your life as a wheel—when one spoke is weak, the ride feels bumpy. The *Happiness Triggers*

11

Wellness Wheel (Figure 1.1) is our guide to building strength in all areas of life.

Figure 1.2 Happiness Triggers Wellness Wheel

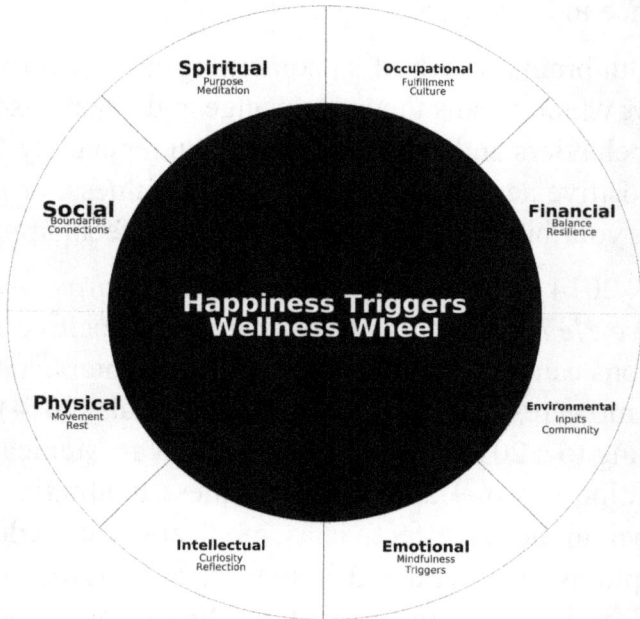

These eight dimensions of wellness; emotional, intellectual, physical, social, spiritual, occupational, financial, and environmental were established by SAMHSA (the Substance Abuse and Mental Health Services Administration) as the foundation for whole-person wellbeing.(SAMHSA, 2016) This book will take you on a journey through each dimension, blending science, storytelling, and practical tools to help you find stability, resilience, and joy.

My Personal Happiness Triggers

Over the years, I've learned what works for me, and I want to share some of my go to Happiness Triggers with you:

1. *Laughter*: Whether it's laughing at my own awkward diabetes moments or watching a funny video, humor instantly boosts my mood.

2. *Movement:* Exercise doesn't always feel like fun at the start, but it works wonders for my mood. Even a short walk or a few pushups on the spot can shift my energy.

3. *Music and Dance:* I'm not the best dancer, but who cares? Cranking up my favorite song and dancing like no one's watching always brings me back to a happier place.

4. *Gratitude:* I used to roll my eyes at the whole "gratitude" thing, but it's a game changer. Taking a minute to focus on what I'm thankful for really shifted my perspective.

5. *Mindfulness:* When life feels overwhelming, mindfulness brings me back to the present moment. It's simple, but powerful.

6. *The Punching Bag:* Sometimes, the best trigger is a little release. I imagine the face of someone who's gotten on my nerves on a punching bag, and let loose. Therapeutic, to say the least.

How to Find Your Own Happiness Triggers

Now it's your turn to create your own happiness toolkit. Here's a fun and simple exercise to help you discover what works best for you.

1. Think of a time when you were really happy. What were you doing? Who were you with? What made that moment special?

2. Write down three things that always lift your mood. It could be anything—your favorite song, food, person, place, or activity.

3. Look at your list. How often do you make time for these things? If it's been a while, think about how you can fit them back into your life.

4. Action Plan: Pick one thing from your list and commit to doing it this week. Start small. Maybe it's as simple as texting a friend who always makes you laugh or listening to a favorite song.

Case Study: Sarah's Story

Let me tell you about Sarah. She was stuck in a rut, overwhelmed by work and family obligations. When I asked her about her Happiness Triggers, she was at a loss. Life has become all about responsibilities.

After some reflection, Sarah remembered she used to love painting. We made a plan: she would spend just 30 minutes a week painting. Fast forward a few weeks, and Sarah's mood had dramatically improved. That small act of reconnecting with something she loved created a ripple effect, making her feel more in control and happier overall.

Simple Mindfulness Exercise: The 54321 Method

You don't need hours of meditation to practice mindfulness. Here's a quick exercise you can do anywhere, anytime you feel overwhelmed.

1. Name 5 things you can see around you.

2. Touch 4 things within reach and notice their texture.

3. Listen for 3 sounds in the background.

4. Smell 2 scents (even if it's just the air around you).

5. Taste 1 thing (take a sip of water or simply notice the taste in your mouth).

This brings you back to the present and calms your mind.

Reflective Exercise: Naming Your Happiness Triggers

Take a few moments to think about your own Happiness Triggers. What are the little things that make you feel better, even on a rough day? Is it hearing your favorite song, grabbing food at a favorite restaurant, or calling someone who always makes you smile?

Journaling Prompt:

Think of a recent moment when you felt stressed or overwhelmed. What Happiness Trigger could you have used to feel better in that moment?

Weekly Challenge: Build Your Happiness Trigger Toolkit

This week, pick one happiness trigger and make it part of your daily routine. Whether it's music, exercise, or humor, use it when you feel your mood slipping. At the end of the week, reflect on how it affected your emotional state.

Final Thoughts — You're In Charge of Your Happiness

Happiness isn't something you need to wait for—it's something you can create. With simple Happiness Triggers like laughter, music, exercise, and mindfulness, you can take control of your emotional state. Even when life gets chaotic, these triggers can help you find joy.

Now it's time…to take action.

What's your next step? Choose a Happiness Trigger and start using it today. The power to create happiness is in your hands.

Chapter 1 References

Cascio, C. N., O'Donnell, M. B., Tinney, F. J., Lieberman, M. D., Taylor, S. E., Strecher, V. J., & Falk, E. B. (2014). Self-affirmation activates brain systems associated with self-related processing and reward and is reinforced by future orientation. *Social Cognitive and Affective Neuroscience*, 11(4), 621-629. doi.org/10.1093/scan/nsv136

Emmons, R. A., & McCullough, M. E. (2003). Counting Blessings Versus Burdens: An Experimental Investigation of Gratitude and Subjective Wellbeing in Daily Life. Journal of Personality and Social Psychology, 84(2), 377389. DOI: 10.1037//0022-3514.84.2.377

Fredrickson, B. L. (2001). The Role of Positive Emotions in Positive Psychology: The Broaden and Build Theory of Positive Emotions. American Psychologist, 56(3), 218226. doi: 10.1037//003-066x.56.3.218

Grossman, P., Niemann, L., Schmidt, S., & Walach, H. (2004). Mindfulness Based Stress Reduction and Health Benefits: A Meta Analysis. *Journal of Psychosomatic Research*, 57(1), 3543. doi: 10.1016/S0022-3999(03)00573-7

Hoge, E. A., Bui, E., Marques, L., Metcalf, C. A., Morris, L. K., Robinaugh, D. J., & Simon, N. M. (2013). Randomized controlled trial of mindfulness meditation for generalized anxiety disorder: Effects on anxiety and stress reactivity. *Journal of the American Medical Association (JAMA)*, 80(3), 171-178. doi.org/10.1001/jamapsychiatry.2013.464

Substance Abuse and Mental Health Services Administration. (2016). Learn the eight dimensions of wellness

[Poster] (Publication No. SMA16-4953). U.S. Department of Health and Human Services. Accessed online July 10, 2025 at https://library.samhsa.gov/product/learn-eight-dimensions-wellness-poster/sma16-4953

Tang, Y.Y., Hölzel, B. K., & Posner, M. I. (2015). The Neuroscience of Mindfulness Meditation. *Nature Reviews Neuroscience*, 16(4), 213225. DOI: 10.1038/nrn3916

Chapter 2. Reinventing Yourself—Embracing the Transformation Journey

Let's Start with a Laugh: Reinventing Myself Like a Broken GPS

Have you ever used a GPS that keeps saying "recalculating" no matter how many times you follow the directions? That's what reinventing yourself can feel like sometimes. You make a plan, think you've got it all figured out, and then life throws you a curveball, leaving you wondering how you ended up in the middle of nowhere. The key is not getting stuck. You just have to laugh, recalculate, and keep moving forward.

Transformation Begins Within

Here's something I've learned: true transformation starts from the inside out. Before you can change anything in your external world, you need to shift your internal world—your mindset, habits, and beliefs. Think of it like upgrading the software before you can enjoy the new features on your device. You can't expect different results if you're running the same old program.

Years before I became the Rev. Dr. Christian Frazier people know today, I had already envisioned myself as a thought leader, author, and mental health advocate. My transformation wasn't about just getting new titles; it was about aligning my inner world with the outer success I was aiming for.

Those Annoying Voices Again

Remember those annoying voices we talked about in Chapter 1? They love to pop up when you're trying to reinvent yourself. You know the ones: "Who do you think you are?" or "You'll never make it." Well, here's what I did: I gave those voices names. Names of people who doubted me. Every time they chimed in, I said, "Shut up, [insert name here], you don't know what you're talking about!" It's empowering. And when they kept coming, I hit them with some affirmations like, "I'm not just enough, I'm MORE than enough."

The Internal Battlefield: Facing Emotional Scars

While the external journey of reinvention is tough, the real battle happens inside. The hardest fights aren't against outside obstacles but the internal struggles—old traumas, self-doubt, and limiting beliefs that rear their ugly heads when you least expect them.

My journey was no different. After leaving the military and entering high-stakes careers in technology and real estate, I was successful on the outside, but inside, I was fighting anxiety and depression. The military had left its scars, and even though I had outward success, the 2008 real estate crash forced me to face my inner demons. This was a turning point. It was clear that external success couldn't fix what was broken inside. That realization marked the beginning of my true transformation.

Reinvention often feels like stripping away layers of armor you've worn for survival. At first, it's uncomfortable—like walking into battle without your shield. But the truth is, the armor we wear to protect ourselves often becomes the very thing that keeps us from growing. For me, shedding that armor meant confronting the fear of failure and admitting that success on paper didn't mean peace in my heart. That's where the real transformation began. Figure 2.1 illustrates this notion of one concept of reinvention.

Figure 2.1 Reinventing Ourself—The Road Ahead

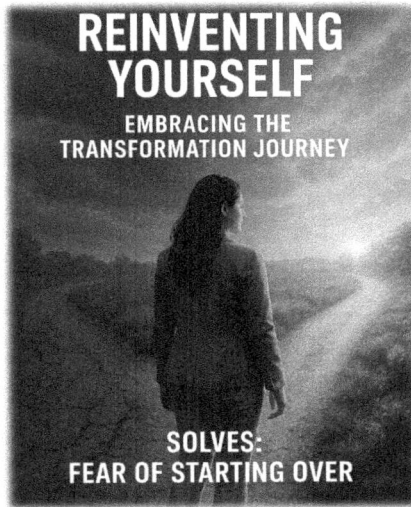

REINVENTING YOURSELF
EMBRACING THE TRANSFORMATION JOURNEY

SOLVES:
FEAR OF STARTING OVER

There is often fear involved in starting over. Whether it is from a relationship that ends, a job transition, moving to a new city, sometimes circumstances can force us to rethink our path or the road we have been on sometimes for years. In these moments we can step back and ask the questions: What's important to us?

What can we do differently?

What steps do we need to take to get to a better place?

The Science of Reinvention: Your Brain on Change

Did you know that your brain is wired to change? Neuroscience backs this up. Thanks to neuroplasticity, your

23

brain can form new connections based on your thoughts and actions.(Doidge, 2007) In other words, you can teach your brain new tricks.

Reinvention isn't just about changing jobs or upgrading your wardrobe; it's about rewiring your brain. Through practices like mindfulness, affirmations, and visualization, you can reshape your brain's pathways to better handle stress, boost confidence, and adopt new habits.

Mindfulness: Staying Present While You Reinvent

One of the best tools I've discovered on my journey of transformation is mindfulness. In 2019, I realized I needed something to help me manage the chaos in my mind, and mindfulness was the answer. Practicing mindfulness helped me become more aware of my thoughts and emotional triggers without judgment.

In fact, mindfulness has been proven to be as effective as medication in treating anxiety, according to a study published in the Journal of the American Medical Association.(Hoge et al., 2023) For me, it became a lifeline. It allowed me to quiet the noise, focus on what really mattered, and stay present in my personal and professional relationships.

Affirmations: Rewriting Your Mental Script

Affirmations are like tiny seeds of positivity that you plant in your brain. According to Sherman and Cohen (2006), self-affirmation helps buffer against stress by affirming core values. Over time, with enough nurturing, they grow into a garden of self-confidence and resilience.

The cool thing is, affirmations actually rewire your brain. A 2019 study in Psychiatry Research showed that affirmations can create long-lasting changes in brain function, helping you develop a more positive mindset. (Shaw & Dobson, 2019) So, the more you tell yourself you're amazing, the more your brain believes it.

Visualization: Seeing Is Believing

If affirmations are the seeds, visualization is the water that helps them grow. Visualization is more than just daydreaming. It's a powerful tool that helps you mentally rehearse your future success. When I started visualizing myself as a confident leader, author, and advocate, my brain started filtering out distractions and focusing on opportunities that matched that vision. Visualization primes the brain to focus on goals by influencing attention and perception.(Ferguson & Bargh, 2004)

Figure 2.2 illustrates the spectrum of issues that can be distractions for us in life. It serves as a reminder of how distractions can be impacts that lead to procrastination and stress that lead to a sense of 'time slipping away from us' in life.

Figure 2.2 Hour Glass Impacts of Distractions

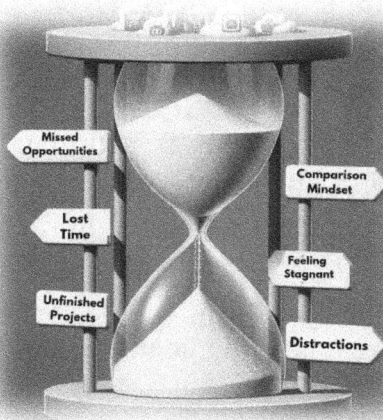

The occurrence of the six topics shown in Figure 2.2 symbolizes the effects of poor time management which can lead to both inefficiency in life generally along with increased stress. This is backed by science too. Visualization helps prime the brain to focus on goals by influencing attention and perception. This mental imagery process can activate cognitive systems that guide our behavior toward achieving desired outcomes, filtering out distractions and honing in on opportunities that align with our goals.(Ferguson & Bargh, 2004) It's like having a built in GPS that keeps recalculating until you reach your destination.

Practical Steps for Reinventing Yourself

Ready to start your transformation journey? Here are some practical steps to get you going:

1. *Challenge Your Paradigms*: Identify the limiting beliefs that are holding you back.

2. *Take Action*: Don't overthink it. Start with small, manageable steps toward your goal.

3. *Address Imposter Syndrome*: It's normal to feel like a fraud when stepping into something new.

4. *Rediscover Your Passions*: Reconnect with what lights you up inside.

5. *Self-Care is Key*: Reinventing yourself takes energy. Eat well, exercise, and get enough rest.

6. *Confront Your Fears*: Fear is a normal part of growth. Facing it builds strength.

7. *Seek Support*: Reinvention is a team sport. Lean on mentors, coaches, or supportive friends.

8. *Redefine Failure*: Treat setbacks as tuition for growth, not proof you can't succeed.

9. *Let Go of Perfectionism*: Progress matters more than perfection.

10. *Embrace Curiosity*: Try new things without needing mastery.

11. *Audit Your Inputs*: Protect your mental diet— monitor what you read, watch, and who you're around.

12. *Build Rituals*: Ground yourself with routines to create momentum and stability.
13. *Track Small Wins*: Keep a victory log to remind yourself of progress.
14. *Serve Others*: Growth accelerates when you help others along their journey.
15. *Celebrate Milestones*: Don't wait until the finish line—celebrate along the way.

Case Study: Ethan's Journey of Reinvention

Ethan was a 42-year-old marketing executive who had everything on paper—great job, high salary, the works. But inside, he felt burned out and empty. He was stuck in imposter syndrome, thinking he wasn't truly good enough despite all his achievements. Ethan decided to make a change. He started practicing mindfulness to quiet his anxious thoughts and began using affirmations to reframe his negative thinking. Slowly but surely, Ethan began to transform. He reignited an old passion for painting and started a side business. While he kept his corporate job, that small shift gave him a renewed sense of purpose and joy.

Reflective Exercises

1. Take 10 minutes to visualize your future self. Imagine the life you want to live, the person you want to

become, and the challenges you'll overcome. Write down the feelings and images that come to mind.

2. Write down three ways you've already reinvented yourself in the past. What did you learn about your resilience from those times?

Journaling Prompt

What limiting beliefs or negative voices have held you back? How can you reframe these beliefs into something more empowering?

Weekly Challenge: Build Your Reinvention Plan

This week, commit to one action that brings you closer to your goals. It could be practicing affirmations, journaling about your future, or facing one of your fears. By the end of the week, reflect on how this step made you feel.

Conclusion — Embrace the Journey

Reinventing yourself isn't about becoming someone else—it's about becoming the best version of yourself. Transformation is a lifelong journey that starts from within. Whether you're changing careers, overcoming obstacles, or just looking for a fresh start, the combination of mindfulness, affirmations, and visualization will help you unlock your true potential.

You have everything you need to create the life you want. Embrace the journey, trust the process, and take that first step today.

Remember, your GPS may keep recalculating, but that's proof you're still moving forward.

Chapter 2 References

Doidge, N. (2007). The brain that changes itself: Stories of personal triumph from the frontiers of brain science. Penguin Random House, LLC.

Ferguson, M. J., & Bargh, J. A. (2004). How social perception can automatically influence behavior. *Trends in Cognitive Sciences, 8*(1), 33–39. https://doi.org/10.1016/j.tics.2003.11.004

Hoge EA, Bui E, Mete M, Dutton MA, Baker AW, Simon NM. (2023). Mindfulness-Based Stress Reduction vs Escitalopram for the Treatment of Adults With Anxiety Disorders: A Randomized Clinical Trial. *JAMA Psychiatry.* 2023;80(1):13–21. doi:10.1001/jamapsychiatry.2022.3679

Shaw, L., & Dobson, K. (2019). The impact of positive affirmations on brain function and emotional regulation: A longitudinal study. *Psychiatry Research, 275*, 102-108. https://doi.org/10.1016/j.psychres.2019.04.003

Sherman, D. K., & Cohen, G. L. (2006). The Psychology of Self Defense: Self Affirmation Theory. *Advances in Experimental Social Psychology,* 38, 183242. https://doi.org/10.1016/S0065-2601(06)38004-5

Chapter 3. The Power of Authenticity – Awakening the True Self Within

Let's Start with a Laugh: Taking the High Road... Well, Most of the Time

So, let me be upfront: I haven't always taken the high road. You know those moments when someone cracks a homophobic joke or throws a slur your way, and you can feel the heat rise in your chest? Yeah, I've been there. I'd love to tell you that I've always responded with mindfulness and calm, but I'd be lying. Sometimes, I've fired back or let it fester, wishing I had said something cleverer or kinder.

But here's the deal: we all have those moments when the pressure to conform or defend ourselves can feel suffocating. For me, it was about suppressing my true self, pretending to be something I wasn't. For you, it might be feeling like you've got to act tough all the time, always be busy, or the one making everyone laugh, like you're being paid to entertain.

We all have our armor—those defenses we put up to navigate the world. But here's the truth: that armor is heavy. Whether it's feeling like you have to be "on" all the time or never showing vulnerability, it takes a toll.

What if we didn't have to wear it all the time? What if we could be... ourselves?

The Struggle to Be True: We All Wear Masks

It doesn't matter who you are, there's a good chance you've put on a mask to fit in at some point in your life. Maybe you've felt like you had to act tough, like there was no room for vulnerability because you had to protect your image. Or maybe you're that person who's always got to be "the life of the party," even when you're exhausted inside. It's like you're constantly performing, but where's your paycheck for all that emotional labor?

I get it. I've worn those masks too. Growing up, I had to suppress my true identity as a gay man because I didn't feel like it fit into the world I was raised in. I became a master of blending in, of being what I thought others wanted me to be. Whether it was in my career or my personal life, I was always editing myself, cutting out the parts I feared others wouldn't accept.

But here's the thing: those masks might help you survive, but they won't help you thrive. They weigh you down, and eventually, they'll crack. Living a life that's out of alignment with who you really are is like running a race with your shoes on the wrong feet, you'll get there, but it's going to hurt, and you'll be way slower than you could've been.

The Cost of Inauthenticity: It's Heavier Than You Think

Here's the tough part: when you're not living authentically, the cost is high. Maybe you feel like you've got to defend your honor every time someone challenges you. Or you've got to be the strong one, the person who never lets anything get to them. Or perhaps you feel like you've got to be busy all the time because slowing down means dealing with your real emotions, and who has time for that, right?

But let me tell you from personal experience, constantly wearing that mask gets exhausting. Whether you're pretending to be something you're not, hiding your emotions, or trying to live up to some impossible standard, it's draining. Over time, it chips away at your mental health. It might look like success from the outside, but on the inside, it feels hollow.

You can't build a fulfilling life on a foundation of inauthenticity. Eventually, something will crack. And when it does, the emotional toll can be overwhelming. Anxiety, depression, burnout, they all come knocking when you've spent too much time pretending to be someone you're not.

My Journey to Authenticity

For years, I lived a double life. On the outside, I was trying to be everything that people expected—a man who fit into the mold. But on the inside, I was suppressing a huge part of myself. I didn't feel like I had room to be vulnerable or to be honest about who I was.

It wasn't until I hit my lowest point—attempting to take my own life—that I realized I couldn't keep living this way. That moment became a turning point for me. I had to start living for myself, not for the expectations of others. I had to take off the mask and let the world see the real me.

It wasn't easy. There were times when being authentic felt scarier than living a lie. But over time, the more I leaned into my truth, the lighter I felt. The weight of pretending fell away, and with it, I gained a sense of freedom that I hadn't known was possible.

Now, I live fully as myself—openly, honestly, and without shame. And you know what? The world didn't fall apart when I did. In fact, my relationships improved. The people who matter stayed, and the ones who didn't... well, they made room for those who love me for who I really am.

The Mental Health Benefits of Authenticity

Here's the good news: living authentically isn't just liberating, it's good for your mental health, too. Studies show that when you live in alignment with your true self, your mental wellbeing improves. (Ryan & Deci, 2017; Wood, et al., 2008) You experience less stress, anxiety, and depression, and more life satisfaction.

When you're not constantly performing or guarding yourself, you can actually breathe. You can focus on what makes you happy instead of what keeps you safe. Living authentically allows you to connect more deeply with others, and most importantly, with yourself.

Practical Exercises to Embrace Authenticity

Ready to take off the mask? Let's work through some exercises to help you reconnect with your true self. You can do these on your own or with someone you trust.

Exercise 1: The Armor List

Grab a piece of paper or open your phone's notes app. Write down all the roles you feel like you "have" to play. Do you feel like you have to be the tough one? The always busy one? The entertainer? Once you've got your list, ask yourself: what would happen if you took off that armor? How would it feel to just be yourself?

Exercise 2: Courageous Conversations

Pick one person in your life with whom you feel comfortable being honest. Share a part of yourself that you've been hiding. It doesn't have to be deep—start small. Maybe it's admitting that you don't love being the life of the party or that you're tired of always being the strong one. Watch how opening up creates space for more authentic connection.

Exercise 3: Find Your Real Joy

Think back to a time when you felt truly happy—when you weren't performing or trying to fit into anyone's mold. What were you doing? Who were you with? Write that down and make a plan to do more of that. It could be painting, taking a long walk, or just hanging out with someone who lets you be 100% yourself.

Exercise 4: Challenge Your Inner Critic

We all have that voice inside our head—the one that says, "You're not good enough," or "You have to be tough all the time." Next time it shows up, challenge it. Ask yourself, "Is this really true? Who taught me to think this way?" Sometimes, just naming that voice helps loosen its grip on you.

Exercise 5: Release Perfection

Authenticity isn't about being perfect. It's about being real. Take one area of your life where you feel the need to be perfect—maybe at work, in your family, or in your friendships—and intentionally let go of that pressure. Allow yourself to be messy, flawed, and human.

Case Study: Maya's Journey to Authenticity

Maya spent years as a lawyer, climbing the corporate ladder and ticking all the boxes for success. But she was miserable. What she really wanted was to be a writer, but she was too afraid of judgment and failure. Eventually, Maya started journaling about her feelings, and through that process, she reconnected with her true passion.

She made the brave decision to leave her law firm and pursue writing full time. The shift wasn't easy, but the more she embraced her true self, the happier and more fulfilled she became. Today, Maya is a successful author and living in alignment with who she really is.

Removing Masks and Discovering Your True Self

For much of our lives, we wear masks—crafted carefully for different audiences. There's the mask we wear at work, polished and professional; the mask we wear with friends, lighthearted and humorous; and the mask we wear with family, perhaps more guarded or dutiful. At first, these masks feel protective, a way to fit in, gain approval, or shield our vulnerabilities. But over time, the weight of wearing multiple masks becomes exhausting. We begin to lose track of who we are beneath them, confusing the performance with our actual identity. Sociologist Erving Goffman described this phenomenon as the "presentation of self," where we act out different roles depending on our audience. (Goffman, 1959) On the surface, this performance helps us fit in, but deep down, it fragments our identity. The question becomes: *Who are we when the stage is empty and the curtain falls?*

The tragedy of masks is that they silence the parts of ourselves yearning for expression. We tell ourselves it's easier to be who people want us to be—more agreeable, more accomplished, more put-together than to reveal the raw, unfiltered truth. Yet authenticity demands that we remove the layers, even when it feels risky. Vulnerability is not weakness; it's the gateway to genuine connection and lasting joy.

This is where the ego comes in. The ego thrives on masks. It identifies itself with what we own, the roles we play, and the labels society gives us. Ego says: *I am my job title. I am my bank account. I am my reputation.* But what happens when those things are stripped away? Who are we without the corner office, the luxury car, the applause, or the curated image on social media? When the masks and ego-driven identities fall away, we are left with a deeper truth: the self that exists beyond accomplishment or approval.

Discovering that self is not about discarding ambition or rejecting success; it's about recognizing that none of those external markers define our essence. Our

39

purpose runs deeper. It is found in the quiet spaces—in how we show up for others, how we cultivate inner peace, and how we contribute to something bigger than ourselves. This journey toward authenticity requires courage, because it often means letting go of the identities that once brought comfort, validation, or status.

And yet, here is the paradox: when we shed the masks and step into authenticity, we actually gain more than we lose. We gain freedom, the freedom to live without constant performance. We gain clarity -the clarity of knowing what truly matters. And we gain connection -the kind of soul-level bonds that can only exist when people meet the real us, not the version we've curated.

The path to authenticity is not a one-time act but a lifelong practice. It requires continual self-reflection and the willingness to ask uncomfortable questions: *Am I living for myself or for approval? Am I speaking my truth or telling people what they want to hear? Am I clinging to an identity because I fear who I might be without it?* These questions can be unsettling, but they are necessary. They strip away the illusions of ego until only the core remains pure, present, and free.

And when we reach that place, something incredible happens. We find our purpose. Purpose doesn't come from masks or ego; it emerges when we align our actions with our deepest values and truths. It is the voice that whispers, even in moments of uncertainty, *This is who you are. This is why you are here.*

Reflective Exercise

Take 10 minutes to journal about the following:

1. List the "masks" you wear in different settings (work, family, friends, community).

2. Write down how each mask makes you feel—does it drain you or energize you?

3. Ask yourself: *If all titles, possessions, and roles were stripped away, who would I still be?*

4. Identify one small step this week where you can show up with fewer masks and more authenticity.

Journaling Prompt

> Where in your life are you putting on a mask to fit in? What's one small step you could take to live more authentically?

Conclusion — The Journey Toward Authenticity

Living authentically isn't about being perfect or having it all figured out. It's about taking off the mask and showing up as you are, flaws and all. It's about recognizing that you're enough, just as you are. And the best part? When you live authentically, you give others permission to do the same. So, take off the armor, stop performing, and let the world see the real you.

Chapter 3 References

Goffman, E. (1956). *The Presentation of Self in Everyday Life*. University of Edinburgh Social Sciences Research Centre. Accessed online August 17, 2025 at https://voidnetwork.gr/wp-content/up-loads/2016/09/The-Presentation-of-Self-in-Everyday-Life-by-Erving-Goffman.pdf

Ryan, R. M., & Deci, E. L. (2017). *Self-determination theory: Basic psychological needs in motivation, development, and wellness.* Guilford Press.

Wood, A. M., Linley, P. A., Maltby, J., Baliousis, M., & Joseph, S. (2008). The authentic personality: A theoretical and empirical conceptualization and the development of the authenticity scale. *Journal of Counseling Psychology, 55*(3), 385-399. https://doi.org/10.1037/0022-0167.55.3.385

Chapter 4. Finding Freedom Beyond the Courtyard—Breaking Free from Mental Prison

Let's Start with a Laugh: Ever Feel Like You're Stuck in Your Own Head?

Have you ever felt trapped in your own mind, like no matter how much progress you make, you're always pulled back into old habits or fears? Maybe you feel like you've always got to be the tough one, showing no signs of vulnerability. Or perhaps you're the life of the party, the one everyone counts on to keep the energy high— even when you're exhausted inside. It's like you're always "on," performing like you should be getting paid for it, but the real paycheck is just burnout.

For me, the mental prison I lived in was about past mistakes and experiences that kept me chained down, even after I'd physically moved on. Whether it was the voice in my head telling me I wasn't good enough or that I had to always be "the strong one," it all felt like I was trapped in my own mind, held back by invisible bars.

You may not have dealt with exactly the same things I have, but we all have our versions of a mental prison.

44

Maybe it's the belief that you're not smart enough, or that you're destined to fail. We've all been there, right? But here's the good news: just like you built that prison, you also hold the key to escape it.

The Mental Prison: How Our Thoughts Keep Us Stuck

Let's be real, many of us live in mental prisons without even realizing it. We're confined by years of negative thinking, self-doubt, and past experiences that hold us back. It's like a record playing the same tune over and over in our heads: "I'm not good enough," "I'll never find love," "I'm not smart enough." Sound familiar?

These limiting beliefs are like the bars of a prison cell, keeping us stuck in the same patterns, unable to break free. The worst part? We often reinforce these beliefs ourselves. It's called confirmation bias—the tendency to only notice things that confirm what we already believe.(Nickerson, 1998; Olejarz, 2017; Soroka, Fournier, & Nir, 2019) So, if you think you're not good enough, you'll focus on every little mistake you make and ignore all the things you do well. It's like putting yourself in solitary confinement, even when there's an open door right in front of you.

Common Mental Prisons

Always needing to be busy: You feel like if you stop, the world will fall apart. Spoiler alert: it won't.

Acting tough all the time: You can't show weakness because someone told you vulnerability was a sign of failure.

Being the life of the party: Everyone expects you to keep the energy up, even when you'd rather be at home in sweatpants binge watching a show.

No room for mistakes: you think one slip up means you've failed, ignoring all your progress along the way.

How Confirmation Bias Keeps Us Locked Up

Think of your brain like a filter. If you believe you're not smart, every time you make a small mistake, your brain says, "See, I told you!" But when you do something right? Your brain conveniently forgets to notice it. This is confirmation bias at work, constantly reinforcing the prison walls around you.

Here's an example: Let's say you've got a belief that you're unlovable. You're in a relationship, and your partner is busy with work. Instead of seeing that they're genuinely caught up, you assume they don't care about you. Why? Because that's what your brain is trained to believe. It becomes a self-fulfilling prophecy, and it keeps you locked in your mental prison.

But what if you could change that filter? What if you could start noticing the good things instead? You can, and that's where Happiness Triggers come in.

Breaking Free from Mental Prisons with Happiness Triggers

The first step to breaking free is realizing that the prison exists in the first place. Once you see it, you can start dismantling it, brick by brick. That's where Happiness Triggers come in. These are simple tools you can use to shift your mindset, break negative thought patterns, and free yourself from the mental chains that hold you back.

Here are some powerful Happiness Triggers that can help you break free:

1. *Gratitude Triggers:* Gratitude is one of the easiest and most effective ways to shift your mindset. When you focus on what you're grateful for, it's like shining a light on all the good in your life, which makes it harder for the darkness to creep in.

    How to Use It: Every morning, write down three things you're grateful for. It could be something small, like a cup of coffee or a friend who makes you laugh. Do this for a week and notice how your perspective starts to change.

2. *Affirmation Triggers:* Affirmations are simple, positive statements that challenge and replace those limiting beliefs. You're essentially telling your brain to shut up and start believing something better.

    How to Use It: Choose an affirmation that speaks to you, like "I am worthy of love" or "I can achieve my goals." Repeat it throughout the day, especially when those negative voices start creeping in.

3. *Meditation Triggers:* Mindfulness and meditation are like a mental reset button. They help you step back, observe your thoughts without judgment, and let go of the ones that aren't serving you.

How to Use It: Spend 10 minutes a day meditating. Focus on your breath, and whenever a negative thought pops up, just acknowledge it and let it pass. No need to dwell on it.

4. *Nature Triggers:* Nature has a magical way of calming the mind. Being outside, even for just a few minutes, can remind you that the world is bigger than your problems.

How to Use It: Take a walk outside, sit by a tree, or just step into your backyard for 10-15 minutes. Let the fresh air and sounds of nature clear your mind.

5. *Music Triggers:* Music can instantly change your mood. Whether it's an upbeat song that makes you want to dance or something calming that helps you relax, music can be a powerful escape from your mental prison.

How to Use It: Create a playlist of songs that lift your spirits. Play it whenever you feel stuck, and let the music shift your energy.

Case Study: Elliot's Journey to Mental Freedom

Elliot was a successful business owner, but despite all his achievements, he felt trapped. He grew up with the belief that financial security was the only measure of success, so he pursued a career in finance, even though his true passion was art. Despite making good money, he felt miserable. He was stuck in a mental prison, believing that if he left finance to pursue art, he'd fail.

Through life coaching, Elliot began to challenge his limiting beliefs. He started using affirmations and practicing mindfulness, slowly dismantling the prison walls he'd built around himself. Over time, he found a balance—pursuing his passion for art while still maintaining financial stability. Today, Elliot is happier than ever, living with the freedom to follow his heart without abandoning his responsibilities.

Reflective Exercise (Solo or with a Partner)

Think about an area of your life where you feel stuck. Is it your career, relationships, or personal goals? Use one of the Happiness Triggers (e.g., gratitude, affirmations, mindfulness) to shift your perspective on that area. If you're doing this with a partner, share your thoughts with them, and talk about how you can both work on breaking free from these limiting beliefs.

Journaling Prompt

What limiting beliefs are keeping you trapped? Write them down, then ask yourself: Are these beliefs really true, or are they just stories I've been telling myself?

Conclusion — Breaking Free is Possible

The walls of your mental prison might feel solid, but they're not. With a little awareness and some powerful Happiness Triggers, you can start to tear those walls down, bit by bit. Remember, the prison exists only in your mind. True freedom comes when you recognize that you hold the key.

So, take a deep breath, step beyond the courtyard of your limiting beliefs, and explore the world that's waiting for you. It's bigger, brighter, and more exciting than you can imagine.

By focusing on the tools that help you break free from your mental prisons, you're not just surviving—you're thriving. Take the steps, use the triggers, and find your way to the freedom you deserve.

Chapter 4 References

Nickerson, R. S. (1998). Confirmation bias: A ubiquitous phenomenon in many guises. *Review of General Psychology, 2*(2), 175–220. https://doi.org/10.1037/1089-2680.2.2.175

Olejarz JM. (July 5, 2017). To Avoid Confirmation Bias in Your Decisions, Consider the Alternatives. *Harvard Business Review Tip.* Accessed online September 28, 2024 at https://hbr.org/tip/2017/07/to-avoid-confirmation-bias-in-your-decisions-consider-the-alternatives

Soroka, S., Fournier, P., & Nir, L. (2019). Negativity bias in news and politics: Antecedents and consequences. *Journal of Communication,* 69(3), 302-324. DOI: 10.1073/pnas.1908369116

Chapter 5. Guarding Your Mind—Rewiring Habits and Fueling Growth

Let's Start with a Thought: Your Mind is a Garden

Imagine your mind as a garden. Whatever seeds you plant will grow. Plant weeds like doubt, fear, and negative thoughts, and you'll end up with a messy, tangled garden that's hard to navigate. But if you plant good seeds—resilience, gratitude, and positivity—you'll watch your life bloom into something beautiful.

The problem is, many of us are unknowingly planting the wrong seeds. It's like trying to grow bananas from peanut seeds. You can't get success, happiness, or personal growth if your mind is stuck in a negative loop. If you're feeding your mind with doubts and fears, you're going to grow more of that negativity. But if you learn to guard your mind and choose what you let in, you can rewire your habits and fuel real growth with an improved mindset.(Dweck, 2006)

Rewiring Bad Habits: The Road to Positive Change

Before we can truly guard our minds, we need to talk about habits. Bad habits aren't just behaviors—they're often the result of years of negative thinking. Maybe it's procrastination, self-doubt, comfort seeking activities like endlessly scrolling on social media, or telling yourself that you're not good enough. These habits become automatic, and before you know it, they're part of your routine.

But here's the good news: your brain is capable of change. Thanks to neuroplasticity, you can form new neural connections and rewire those bad habits into healthier ones.(May, 2011; Kolb & Gibb, 2011)

How to Start Rewiring Bad Habits

1. *Identify Your Habit Triggers*: Every habit starts with a trigger. For example, you feel stressed (trigger), so you binge watch TV (routine), and you feel temporary relief (reward). To break the cycle, identify the trigger and replace the routine with something positive—like going for a short walk or practicing deep breathing. Over time, your brain will associate the new routine with the reward, creating a healthier habit.

2. *Activate Happiness Triggers*: Introducing Happiness Triggers into your routine can help you replace bad habits. For example, if you're caught in negative

thinking, take a moment to list three things you're grateful for. This simple shift rewires your brain for positivity. Affirmations also help—repeating phrases like "I am capable of change" or "I'm getting stronger every day" will break the negative thought patterns.

3. *Track Your Progress*: Change doesn't happen overnight, but tracking your progress makes it easier. Keep a habit tracker or journal and note every time you replace a bad habit with a positive one. Over time, these small wins add up and motivate you to keep going.

Guarding Your Mind in a Hyperconnected World

We live in a world where we're bombarded with information every minute of the day. From social media to news updates, it's easy to get overwhelmed.(Soroka, Fournier, & Nir, 2019) If we're not careful, this mental clutter can cloud our thoughts and hold us back.

Think of your mind like your body—just as you wouldn't eat junk food all day and expect to feel healthy, you can't let mental junk in and expect to grow. The key is to filter out what doesn't serve you.

1. *Choose Content That Inspires Growth*: Not all content is created equal. Sure, a good Netflix binge is fun, but it's important to balance that with content that helps you grow. Choose podcasts, books, or videos that challenge your thinking and expand your knowledge. Focus on things that help you become the person you want to be.

2. *Limit Negative Inputs*: Social media is a breeding ground for comparison, negativity, and self-doubt. If you feel drained after scrolling, it's time to declutter your feed. Unfollow accounts that bring you down and replace them with ones that inspire or uplift you.

3. *Track Your Content Consumption*: Be mindful of how much time you're spending consuming different forms of media. Ask yourself: Is this making me feel better or worse? Reflect on how it affects your mood and take action to cut out the stuff that doesn't serve you.

Building a Supportive Environment for Growth

Just like the content you consume, the people you surround yourself with have a big impact on your mindset. If you're surrounded by negative influences, it's going to be a lot harder to stay positive and grow.

Creating a Growth Focused Environment

1. *Family and Friends*: Be open with your loved ones about your goals and challenges. While not everyone will understand your journey, that's okay. Focus on surrounding yourself with people who support and encourage your growth.

2. *Seek Mentors or Coaches*: Sometimes, we all need a little guidance. Whether it's a mentor, life coach, or therapist, having someone who has walked the path before can provide invaluable advice and help you overcome mental barriers.

Stepping Outside Your Comfort Zone: The Path to Growth

Growth comes from discomfort. If you stay in your comfort zone, you're not going to grow. It's only when you step into new, challenging situations that you start to see real change.

How to Step Out of Your Comfort Zone

1. *Set Learning Intentions*: Whether you're attending a workshop, reading a book, or starting a new hobby, set clear goals. What do you hope to learn? How will this help you grow? Being intentional about your learning ensures you get the most out of every experience.

2. *Celebrate Your Wins*: Growth is a process, and it's important to celebrate your progress along the way. Whether it's a small win like finishing a book or a big win like landing a new job, take time to acknowledge and celebrate your efforts.

3. *Turn Entertainment into Education*: Who says learning can't be fun? Choose movies, documentaries, or shows that offer valuable life lessons, resilience stories, or insights into personal growth. Turn entertainment into a tool for growth.

Happiness Triggers for Rewiring Habits

Incorporating Happiness Triggers into your daily routine can make all the difference. Here's how they can help:

1. *Affirmations for Confidence*: Positive affirmations help you shift your mindset when things get tough. Try repeating affirmations like, "I am becoming stronger every day," or "I am more than capable." These simple statements reinforce a growth mindset and help you stay focused.

2. *Gratitude for Perspective*: Gratitude is like a magic switch that shifts your focus from what you don't have to what you do. Start your day by listing three things you're grateful for. This habit rewires your brain to see challenges as opportunities instead of obstacles.

Case Study: Breaking the Digital Overload

Let's talk about Sarah, a marketing professional who felt completely overwhelmed. She was spending hours every day scrolling through social media, but instead of feeling inspired, she felt drained. It wasn't just time wasted—it was her mental energy being sucked into comparison and negativity.

Sarah decided to take control of her content consumption. She tracked how much time she was spending on social media and realized it was nearly two hours a day! So, she made a plan: she replaced her scrolling time with activities that nurtured her growth, like reading, listening to podcasts, and spending time outside.

After just a few months, Sarah's mindset had transformed. She was less anxious, more focused, and filled with positive energy. By guarding her mind and curating a growth focused environment, she rewired her habits and found a sense of peace and productivity she hadn't felt in years.

Reflective Exercise (Do It Solo or With a Partner)

Track your content consumption for a week. Write down how much time you spend on social media, watching TV, or scrolling the news. Reflect on how it made you feel—energized or drained? What changes can you make to guard your mind better?

Tip: If you're doing this with a partner, compare notes and support each other in making positive changes.

Journaling Prompt

> What influences your thoughts and habits? Take a look at what you consume daily—social media, TV, conversations. What is lifting you up, and what's dragging you down? How can you start focusing on more positive inputs?

Conclusion — You Control the Garden of Your Mind

Your mind is like a garden, and what you plant is what will grow. If you want to grow a healthy, thriving life, you need to guard your mind carefully. Choose positive inputs, track your habits, and activate Happiness Triggers to rewire your mindset and fuel your growth.

Remember, you can't expect apples from orange seeds. What you think, feel, and believe directly impacts your results. So, plant resilience, gratitude, and positivity, and watch your life bloom into something amazing.

By guarding your mind, rewiring your habits, and focusing on growth, you're paving the way for a future filled with success and happiness. Keep planting those good seeds!

Chapter 5 References

Dweck, C. S. (2006). Mindset: The New Psychology of Success. Ballantine Books.

Kolb, B., & Gibb, R.(2011). Brain plasticity and behaviour in the developing brain. *Journal of the Canadian Academy of Child and Adolescent Psychiatry*, 20(4), 265-276.

May, A. (2011). Experience-dependent structural plasticity in the adult human brain. *Trends in Cognitive Sciences*, 15(10), 475-482. https://doi.org/10.1016/j.tics.2011.08.002

Soroka, S., Fournier, P., & Nir, L. (2019). Cross-national evidence of a negativity bias in psychophysiological reactions to news. *Proceedings of the National Academy of Sciences of the United States of America*, 116(38),18888–18892. https://doi.org/10.1073/pnas.1908369116

Chapter 6. Fueling Happiness—The Power of Exercise and Nutrition Triggers for a Healthier Mind

Let's start with the obvious: we all want to feel good, right? But did you know that feeling great doesn't just come from thinking positively or being around happy people? A huge part of your happiness comes from how you treat your body. That's right—your physical health and mental wellbeing are best buddies, and they work together to keep you in a good mood.(Kim & Johnson, 2019)

Rev. Dr. Christian Frazier is living proof of this. After shedding significant weight and being featured on the front page of the New York Post, my story became one of transformation, not just physically, but mentally as well. Through better eating and regular exercise, I found more energy, better sleep, and less reliance on medications. If a busy guy like me can make these changes, so can you!

So, let's dive into how simple things like moving your body and eating well can be powerful Happiness Triggers.

Why Exercise Equals Happiness

Exercise isn't just about getting buff or fitting into your old jeans (though, hey, that's a nice bonus). It's actually a fantastic way to boost your mood. You've probably heard about endorphins—those "feelgood" chemicals your body releases when you move. They're like nature's free antidepressants, lifting your spirits and helping reduce stress, anxiety, and depression. In fact, some studies suggest that regular exercise can be just as effective as medication for mild to moderate depression.

But here's the kicker: it's not just about those feel good chemicals. Exercise gives you a sense of accomplishment. Whether you're crushing a new fitness goal or just making time to go for a walk, you build confidence every time you move. This isn't just about physical health—it's about proving to yourself that you're capable of change and growth.

My personal story shows this firsthand. By making exercise part of my daily routine, I didn't just lose weight—he gained energy, clarity, and freedom from medications. It's not about doing hours at the gym, it's about finding something you enjoy and sticking with it.

How Exercise Triggers Work

So, how exactly does exercise act as a Happiness Trigger? Simple: it distracts you from worries and helps you focus on the present. Whether you're lifting weights, walking, or dancing in your living room, exercise pulls your mind away from stress and puts it into the moment. It's like giving your brain a much-needed break.

And it's not just solo work. Exercise can also be social. Ever tried a fitness class or played a team sport? Moving with others not only helps you stay motivated but also builds a sense of community, and having good people around you is one of the best ways to keep your mood up.

Easy Ways to Add Exercise to Your Routine

You don't have to start training for a marathon to feel the benefits of exercise. In fact, you can get a happiness boost from something as simple as walking. The key is to do what feels good to you—if dancing around your house makes you happy, go for it!

Here are a few ideas:

1. *Walk and Talk*: Next time you catch up with a friend, do it while walking. It's a great way to combine movement with connection.

2. *Sneaky Exercise*: Take the stairs instead of the elevator, park farther away, or even do some stretches during TV commercials.

3. *Find Your Fun*: Love music? Try a dance class. Like being outdoors? Go for a hike. The point is to enjoy what you're doing so it becomes part of your life, not just a chore.

4. *The GutBrain Connection*: You Are What You Eat (Literally)

We've all heard the phrase "You are what you eat," but it's especially true when it comes to your mental health. There's something called the gut brain connection, which means that what you put in your body can either help or hurt your mental wellbeing.(Naidoo, 2020)

Think of your gut as a second brain. It's full of neurons that communicate directly with your actual brain, which is why your diet can affect your mood, focus, and even anxiety levels. If you're filling up on junk food, your gut bacteria get out of whack, and that can lead to feeling sluggish, irritable, or anxious.

But when you focus on whole foods—fruits, vegetables, lean proteins, and healthy fats—you're not just fueling your body, you're also fueling your mind. These foods keep your gut happy and help balance the chemicals in your brain that regulate mood.

How to Use Nutrition as a Happiness Trigger

If the idea of changing your diet seems overwhelming, don't worry—it doesn't have to be complicated. Poor diet and lack of physical activity can contribute to chronic inflammation, which negatively affects mental health.(Dantzer et al., 2008) Inflammation in the body, caused by poor lifestyle choices such as a diet high in processed foods and a sedentary lifestyle, is linked to mental health issues like depression and anxiety.(Firth et al., 2020)

Here's how you can start using nutrition to boost your happiness:

1. *Eat Real Food*: Stick to whole foods like veggies, fruits, nuts, and lean proteins. These give your body and brain what they need to function at their best.

2. *Cut Back on the Junk*: Processed foods and sugar mess with your gut and brain connection, leading to mood swings and fatigue. Start by cutting back a little each day and replacing junk with healthier choices.

3. *Pay Attention*: Notice how you feel after eating different foods. Do you feel energized after a salad but tired after fast food? Your body is always sending signals—listen to them!

4. *Tracking Progress*: The Secret to Staying on Track.

It's easy to fall off the wagon when trying to make new changes. That's why keeping track of what you eat and how you move is so helpful. You don't have to be obsessive about it, but even a simple journal can show you patterns and help you stay motivated.

1. *Wellness Journal*: Write down what you ate, how much you moved, and how you felt each day. Over time, you'll see what foods or activities give you the most energy and happiness.

2. *Track Your Sleep and Stress*: Better food and more movement usually lead to better sleep. Keep an eye on how your new habits are affecting your sleep quality and stress levels.

Case Study: Marcus' Journey to Better Health

Take Marcus, a 45-year-old dad who was always tired, stressed, and not sleeping well. He wasn't exercising much, and his diet was filled with processed snacks and takeout meals. He decided to make a change, starting with a daily walk and swapping junk food for healthier options.

Marcus started tracking his progress in a journal, noting that after just a week, he had more energy and was sleeping better. Over time, these small changes added up. Marcus felt happier, less stressed, and more in control of his life. His story is proof that taking care of your body has a direct effect on your mind.

Reflective Exercise (Do It Solo or With a Partner)

Track your meals and physical activity for one week. After each meal or workout, write down how you felt—did it give you more energy? Did it make you feel sluggish? At the end of the week, review your notes and see if you notice any patterns. If you're doing this with a partner, compare your experiences and encourage each other to keep going!

Journaling Prompt

> How do your current eating habits and activity levels make you feel? What small changes could you make to feel better both physically and mentally?

Conclusion — Move Your Body, Feed Your Mind

Your body and mind are a team, and when you take care of one, you're helping the other. By adding more movement and making smarter food choices, you'll not only feel better physically, but your mental health will improve, too.

Start small. Move more, eat better, and pay attention to how these changes make you feel. You'll be surprised at how even small shifts can lead to big improvements in your happiness and wellbeing.

Chapter 6 References

Dantzer, R., O'Connor, J. C., Freund, G. G., Johnson, R. W., & Kelley, K. W. (2008). From inflammation to sickness and depression: When the immune system subjugates the brain. *Nature Reviews Neuroscience, 9*(1), 46-56. https://doi.org/10.1038/nrn2297

Naidoo, U. (2020). Gut feelings: How food affects your mood. *Harvard Health Blog.* Accessed online October 17, 2024 at https://www.health.harvard.edu/blog/gut-feelings-how-food-affects-your-mood-2018120715548

Kim, S., & Johnson, T. (2019). The role of exercise and nutrition in boosting mental well-being. *The Journal of Positive Psychology, 14*(4), 310-320. https://doi.org/10.1080/17439760.2019.1579351

Firth, J., Gangwisch, J. E., Borsini, A., Wootton, R. E., & Mayer, E. A. (2020). Food and mood: How do diet and nutrition affect mental wellbeing? *BMJ, 369,* m2382. https://doi.org/10.1136/bmj.m2382

Chapter 7. The Power of Letting Go and Building Resilience

Introduction: Freeing Yourself from the Weight of the Past

Throughout life, we accumulate experiences—some uplifting, others painful. The emotional baggage from past hurts, resentments, and anger can weigh heavily on our well-being, holding us back from achieving true happiness. Many people feel they need to hold on to these negative emotions as a form of self-protection or validation of their experiences. However, research shows that releasing these burdens is one of the most powerful acts of self-love and resilience.

Holding onto anger and resentment is like carrying a heavy backpack filled with stones; it drains our energy and hinders personal growth. Learning to let go isn't about erasing memories or dismissing experiences; rather, it's a journey of self-compassion and empowerment, allowing us to reclaim control over our own happiness. This chapter will explore techniques for releasing anger and resentment, building emotional resilience, and embracing forgiveness, ultimately creating space for peace and joy.

The Science Behind Letting Go and Resilience

Studies indicate that unresolved anger and resentment are associated with increased cortisol levels, leading to stress and health issues.(Harris & Thompson, 2017) On the other hand, practicing forgiveness and gratitude can reduce stress hormones and promote a healthier mindset. According to research, forgiveness is not only beneficial for emotional well-being but can also significantly improve physical health, reducing the risk of heart disease and lowering blood pressure.(Fredrickson, 2001)

This figure highlights several examples noted in the chapter that can embody resentments, grudges, or past traumas that can weigh us down emotionally. From my own life experience the image symbolizes someone carrying a heavy backpack filled with all this emotional baggage is intended to give you a visual that you can apply to remembering the importance of letting go of some of these issues in life.

Why We Hold on and How It Affects Us

Why is it so difficult to let go of anger? Anger often feels justified, especially when we've been wronged. We may believe that holding onto these feelings protects us from future harm. However, in reality, these negative emotions keep us trapped in the past, making it difficult to move forward. Over time, holding onto resentment can lead to emotional exhaustion and de-creased overall happiness.

Techniques for Releasing Anger and Resentment

1. *Mindfulness Meditation*:

Mindfulness teaches us to observe our thoughts and feelings without judgment, allowing us to acknowledge emotions like anger without letting them define us. By practicing mindfulness, we develop a greater awareness of our thoughts and learn to let go of those that no longer serve us.

Mindfulness Exercise for Letting Go

- Find a quiet space and sit comfortably. Close your eyes and take several deep breaths.
- Bring to mind a situation or person that has caused you pain.
- As you breathe in, acknowledge the pain and tension. As you exhale, visualize releasing that tension.
- Repeat for 5–10 minutes, allowing yourself to let go a little more with each breath.

This practice not only reduces stress but also creates mental space to reframe negative experiences from a place of compassion rather than anger.

2. *Practicing Forgiveness*:

Forgiveness is a powerful tool for emotional freedom. Research shows that forgiveness releases us from the emotional grip of past hurt and empowers us to move forward with resilience.(Emmons & McCullough, 2003) Forgiveness doesn't mean forgetting or condoning harm but choosing to release the anger associated with it.

Visualization Exercise for Forgiveness

- Close your eyes and imagine the person who caused you pain.

- Picture them surrounded by a warm light and acknowledge their humanity.

- Silently repeat the phrase: "I forgive you for my own peace and healing."

- Practice this daily for a week, gradually allowing the weight of resentment to lift.

3. *Affirmations for Emotional Release*

Affirmations are a powerful way to reprogram our mindset and encourage emotional release. Positive affirmations can help redirect our focus from pain to peace, allowing us to move forward without anger.

Affirmations for Letting Go

- "I release my past and open my heart to peace and love."

- "Forgiveness sets me free and fills me with peace."

- "I am no longer defined by my pain. I am stronger and more resilient."

Repeating these affirmations daily reinforces the mindset shift necessary to move from resentment to compassion, building resilience in the process.

4. *Journaling for Reflection and Clarity*:

Writing down our thoughts is a powerful way to process emotions and gain clarity. Journaling allows us to put our experiences into words, helping to release trapped feelings and promote a sense of emotional resolution.

Journaling Exercise: Release and Renew

- Take a blank page and write down everything you feel about a situation or person that has hurt you.

- Be honest, letting every emotion flow onto the paper.

- After you've finished, write a closing statement: "I release this for my own peace and healing."

- Tear up the page or safely burn it as a symbolic act of release.

This exercise allows you to confront your feelings in a safe space, promoting catharsis and reinforcing the power of letting go.

Building Resilience: A Path Forward

Resilience is the ability to bounce back from adversity, and it is cultivated by consistently choosing to let go of what no longer serves us. Letting go creates room for resilience to flourish, as it allows us to detach from the past and focus on growth. Building resilience requires daily practices, like gratitude and mindfulness, that reinforce our ability to move forward despite challenges.

Daily Practices to Reinforce Resilience

1. *Gratitude Practice*: Start each day by listing three things you are grateful for. This helps shift focus from pain to positivity.
2. *Daily Mindfulness*: Spend five minutes each morning focused on your breathing. This anchors you in the present moment and reduces stress.
3. *Acts of Kindness*: Helping others can lift your mood and build resilience by reinforcing the interconnectedness of our experiences.

Case Study: Marcus's Journey to Resilience

In this chapter, we revisit Marcus, a man whose life was shaped by betrayal from a close friend. For years, Marcus felt unable to release his anger, replaying the situation repeatedly, which led to emotional exhaustion and anxiety. Despite the encouragement of friends and family, Marcus struggled to let go, fearing that forgiving would mean condoning the betrayal.

Through his mindfulness journey, Marcus began using visualization exercises and daily affirmations, as well as practicing gratitude. Slowly, he noticed his focus shifting from anger toward compassion and inner peace. Marcus began journaling, reflecting on his values and the kind of person he wanted to become. In the process, he released his resentment, feeling more at peace and resilient.

Purpose of Case Study: This case study illustrates how real-life application of mindfulness, forgiveness, and resilience techniques can lead to personal transformation, encouraging readers to relate Marcus's journey to their own lives.

Reflective Exercises

Exercise 1: Exploring Resentment and Its Effects

- Take a few minutes to close your eyes, focus on your breathing, and bring to mind a past event or person that triggers feelings of resentment.

- Reflect on how these feelings have impacted different aspects of your life—emotionally, mentally, and even physically.

- Ask yourself, "What would my life look like if I released this resentment? How would it free up my energy and focus?"

Purpose: This reflection encourages a deeper understanding of how lingering negative emotions like resentment affect our well-being, helping you visualize the benefits of letting got.

Exercise 2: Practicing Forgiveness as a Path to Freedom

- Think of a recent moment when you felt hurt, angered, or let down. Try to see the situation from the other person's perspective, recognizing their humanity.

- Reflect on the following: "What aspects of this experience do I have the power to release for my own peace?"

- Visualize yourself forgiving this person or situation, not for their sake, but to reclaim your own happiness and resilience.

Purpose: This exercise is designed to reframe forgiveness as an act of self-compassion and empowerment, helping you realize the control you have over your emotional well-being.

Journaling Prompts

Prompt 1: Unpacking Anger and Resentment

- Write about a situation in your life where you still feel anger or resentment. Describe the event in detail, as well as the emotions it evokes.

- Now, ask yourself, "What have I learned from this experience? How can I move forward without carrying this weight?"

- Reflect on how you might reframe this experience to focus on personal growth rather than the pain it initially caused.

Purpose: This prompt helps process negative emotions, encouraging you to understand and eventually release resentment by focusing on the lessons learned.

Prompt 2: A Letter of Forgiveness

- Write a letter to yourself or someone else who has caused you pain. Express the impact this experience had on you, both positively and negatively.

- End the letter by acknowledging your decision to forgive, whether partially or fully, as a means of releasing your own emotional burdens.

- Consider keeping this letter as a reminder of your commitment to let go, or safely dispose of it as a symbolic release.

Purpose: Writing a letter of forgiveness can be a cathartic exercise that solidifies the decision to let go, creating a tangible sense of closure.

Conclusion — The Gift of Forgiveness

Forgiveness is the greatest gift you can give yourself. It's not about letting someone else off the hook—it's about freeing yourself from the emotional baggage that's been weighing you down. By choosing to forgive, you open yourself up to peace, healing, and the possibility of happiness. So let go of the past, drop the heavy load, and finally feel the relief that comes from setting yourself free.

Letting go of unforgiveness is one of the most powerful acts of self-love you can offer yourself. Remember, it's not about excusing someone's actions—it's about freeing yourself from the weight that's holding you back.

Chapter 7 References

Emmons, R. A., & McCullough, M. E. (2003). Counting blessings versus burdens: An experimental investigation of gratitude and subjective well-being in daily life. *Journal of Personality and Social Psychology*, 84(2), 377-389. https://doi.org/10.1037/0022-3514.84.2.377

Fredrickson, B. L. (2001). The role of positive emotions in positive psychology: The broaden-and-build theory of positive emotions. *American Psychologist*, 56(3), 218-226. https://doi.org/10.1037/003-066X.56.3.218

Harris, L. J., & Thompson, E. P. (2017). How practicing gratitude rewires the brain for positivity. *The Journal of Positive Psychology*, 12(5), 460–472. https://doi.org/10.1080/17439760.2016.1227334

Chapter 8. The Healing Power of Creative Expression

Let's be honest: life can be overwhelming, stressful, and downright exhausting. But what if there was a way to channel all that stress and emotion into something positive—something that makes you feel lighter, freer, and happier? That's where creative expression comes in. Whether it's through singing, painting, dancing, or writing, tapping into your creative side can be a powerful way to process emotions, heal, and, most importantly, rediscover your joy.

In this chapter, we're going to explore how creative outlets can be Happiness Triggers—simple, enjoyable activities that instantly lift your mood and help you work through emotional challenges. And don't worry— you don't need to be Picasso or Beyoncé to benefit from creative expression. This is about freedom, not perfection.

The Science Behind Creative Expression

Ever get so lost in an activity that time seems to disappear? That's called "flow," a state where you're so immersed in what you're doing that everything else fades away. Psychologist Mihaly Csikszentmihalyi coined the term, and studies show that people who experience flow regularly are happier, more fulfilled, and even healthier.(Csikszentmihalyi, 1990)

When you engage in creative activities like painting, singing, or dancing, your brain's reward system kicks in, releasing dopamine—the feel-good chemical. This helps reduce anxiety, stress, and symptoms of depression, all while boosting your sense of satisfaction.(Van Der Kolk, 2014; Csikszentmihalyi, 1997)

Essentially, creativity isn't just fun; it's good for your brain and your emotional wellbeing.

Breaking Through Creative Blocks

Staring at a blank page can feel like your brain has gone on strike. The cursor blinks, the ideas hide, and suddenly you're convinced you've lost your creative spark. Here's the truth: every creative—authors, musicians, inventors—hits this wall. Writer's block isn't a sign that you're broken; it's often a sign that your mind needs a reset.

Why Creative Blocks Happen

Blocks usually come from one of three sources:

- **Perfectionism** – the fear of not writing it "right."
- **Exhaustion** – burnout from pushing too hard.

- **Fear of Judgment** – worrying about what others will think.

Science shows that creativity thrives when the brain's "default mode network" is allowed to wander.(Beaty et al., 2015) In other words, giving your mind space can actually lead to breakthroughs.

My Own Creative Blocks

When I was writing *Happiness Triggers*, I hit walls too. There were days when the words wouldn't flow, especially during the five months I was living in a hotel after the hurricane. But I learned that blocks don't mean stop—they mean pause, breathe, and try a different route.

Grounding to Reset Creativity: The 4-7-8 Method

One tool I used often was the **4-7-8 breathing method**. Here's how it works:

1. Inhale through your nose for 4 seconds.

2. Hold your breath for 7 seconds.

3. Exhale slowly through your mouth for 8 seconds.

4. Repeat for four cycles.

This quick reset lowers anxiety, oxygenates your brain, and creates space for new ideas to surface. More than once, I found clarity right after a round of 4-7-8 breathing.

Practical Tools to Beat Creative Blocks

Here are strategies you can apply the next time you feel stuck:

1. **Freewrite:** Put pen to paper and write without stopping for 10 minutes—even if it's nonsense. It loosens your creative muscles.

2. **Change Your Environment:** Move to a new spot, even for 15 minutes. A fresh setting sparks fresh thoughts.

3. **Micro-Goals:** Instead of "finish the chapter," commit to "write 5 sentences." Small wins build momentum.

4. **Creative Cross-Training:** Try drawing, playing music, or even cooking—other creative outlets unlock different brain pathways.

5. **Step Away:** Give your brain incubation time. Sometimes the best ideas come in the shower, on a walk, or while driving.

6. **Use Prompts:** Answer a reflective question related to your theme. Prompts break the pressure of "creating from nothing."

7. **Accountability:** Share your progress with a trusted friend or mentor. Being seen often pulls you out of hiding.

Reflective Exercise

Next time you feel blocked, pause for 4-7-8 breathing, then freewrite one messy paragraph. Ask yourself: *What am I afraid to put on this page?* Often, naming the fear unlocks the flow.

Closing Thought on Creative Blocks

Creative blocks are not barriers—they are bridges. They remind you to pause, reset, and find a new way through. Every time you break through a block, you strengthen not just your writing, but your resilience.

Pathways for Opening Your Creative Voice

Creativity often feels like a spark out of nowhere, but neuroscience shows it's more like a symphony than a lightning bolt. When we are at our most creative, the brain isn't chaotic—it's orchestrating a balance between imagination and control. The *default mode network* (linked to daydreaming and free association) collaborates with the *executive control network* (responsible for focus and decision-making).

This dynamic interplay is what allows breakthroughs to emerge—not from pure chaos or rigid structure, but from their integration.(Beaty et al., 2015) Additionally, researchers in the field of creativity studies have long emphasized that innovation is not about sudden genius but about deliberate practice, openness to experience, and persistence over time.(Kaufman & Beghetto, 2009) In other words, creativity is not just a gift—it's a skill set we can strengthen, a muscle that grows when we engage with it intentionally. The next four subtopics offer ideas on ways to unleash your own creative expression.

Singing: Letting Your Voice Be Free

You don't need to be a professional singer to enjoy the benefits of singing. Whether you're belting it out in the shower or singing along to your favorite playlist in the car, singing can be a powerful emotional release. Research shows that singing releases endorphins and oxytocin, which lower stress and improve mood. Plus, it helps regulate your breathing, which calms your nervous system.(Fancourt et al., 2016; Kreutz et al., 2004)

Next time you're feeling down, give it a try. Sing your favorite song out loud—it doesn't matter if you hit the right notes. You'll feel lighter, more relaxed, and maybe even a little silly (in a good way). Singing is one of the simplest ways to engage in creative expression, and you can do it anywhere.

Writing and Poetry: Giving Words to Your Emotions

If you've ever journaled after a tough day or written down your thoughts when you couldn't sleep, you know how powerful writing can be. Expressive writing, like journaling or poetry, allows you to give voice to feelings that might otherwise stay bottled up. It helps you reflect, process, and ultimately release what's been weighing you down.

Spoken word poetry takes it to another level by combining the power of words with the freedom of performance. It's not just about writing—it's about telling your story. And the beauty of it? You don't have to share it with anyone if you don't want to. Writing is a deeply personal way to explore your thoughts and emotions, and it offers a unique opportunity for healing.

Dancing: Moving Through Emotions

Feeling stressed? Put on your favorite song and dance like nobody's watching. Dance is one of the most primal forms of creative expression, allowing you to release emotions through movement. Whether you're grooving to a beat in your living room or taking a dance class, moving your body helps reduce stress, boosts your mood, and connects you to your physical self.

You don't need fancy choreography or years of training to benefit from dance. In fact, studies show that even simple, spontaneous dancing can reduce symptoms of anxiety and depression. Just let go, move however you want, and enjoy the freedom that comes with it.

Art: The Power of Visual Expression

Sometimes, words aren't enough to express what's going on inside. That's where art comes in. Whether you're painting, drawing, or doodling, visual art offers a way to communicate emotions that are hard to put into words. You don't need to be an artist to benefit from creating—it's about the process, not the outcome.

A study from the *International Journal of Offender Therapy Comparative Criminology* found that engaging in art helped participants lower their stress levels and improve their mood.(Gussak, 2007) It's about giving yourself permission to explore your feelings through color, shape, and texture, creating something that's uniquely yours. Art becomes a visual language of healing, where your emotions can flow freely onto the canvas.

Why Creative Expression Is Essential for Mental Health

Here's why making time for creative activities can significantly improve your mental wellbeing:

1. *Reduces Stress and Anxiety*: Creativity calms the mind and body. Whether you're singing, drawing, or dancing, creative expression helps bring you into the present moment, which is a powerful antidote to stress.

2. *Builds Emotional Resilience*: Creative outlets help you process emotions, rather than suppressing them.

When you engage in creative activities, you're able to release difficult emotions like anger, sadness, or frustration in a healthy way.

3. *Promotes Self Discovery*: Creative expression helps you tap into parts of yourself that you may not have known were there. It's a way of exploring your identity, emotions, and dreams in a safe and constructive way.

4. *Fosters Connection*: Sharing your creative work—whether it's a poem, a painting, or a song—can help you connect with others. Creative expression can deepen relationships by helping others understand your inner world.

Simple Ways to Add Creative Expression to Your Life

Here are some easy, fun ways to make creative expression a part of your daily routine:

1. *Start a Journal:* Set aside just 10 minutes a day to write about your thoughts and feelings. Don't worry about making it perfect—just let your words flow freely.

2. *Sing Every Day:* Whether it's humming in the kitchen or singing your heart out in the shower, make singing a part of your daily life. It's a simple way to lift your spirits.

3. *Dance It Out:* You don't need a dance floor—your living room will do just fine! Put on a song you love and dance without worrying about how you look. Just enjoy the movement.

4. *Create Art:* Try doodling, painting, or even coloring in a coloring book. Art is a great way to express yourself visually and can be incredibly therapeutic.

5. *Write Poetry or Spoken Word:* Don't be afraid to put your feelings into words. Try writing a poem about something you're going through, and if you're feeling bold, share it aloud.

Case Study: The Healing Power of Creative Expression

Jasmine, a 28-year-old artist, found herself struggling with anxiety and grief after losing a family member. Traditional therapy helped, but it wasn't until she started painting that she felt a true release. Art became her way of processing the deep emotions she couldn't express with words. Over time, Jasmine noticed that painting not only improved her mood but also allowed her to feel more connected to herself. Her creative practice became her personal sanctuary.

Reflective Exercise (Do It Alone or With a Friend)

Spend 15 minutes today engaging in a creative activity. It could be anything—singing, dancing, writing, or drawing. Afterward, write down how the activity made you feel. If you're doing this exercise with a friend, share your creative work and talk about the emotions it brought up.

Journaling Prompt

> What creative activities have made you feel happy in the past? How can you bring more of these activities into your life now? How do you feel when you express yourself creatively?

Conclusion — The Journey of Creativity and Healing

Creative expression is about freedom, not perfection. It's a way to tap into your inner self, release your emotions, and find joy in the process. Whether you're singing in the car, doodling in a notebook, or dancing in your living room, let your creativity lead you toward healing and happiness.

So, take that first step. Grab a paintbrush, hum a tune, or start a journal. Let your creative spirit guide you toward greater happiness and inner peace. After all, creativity is a powerful tool for healing—and it's always within your reach.

Chapter 8 References

Beaty, R. E., Benedek, M., Silvia, P. J., & Schacter, D. L. (2015). Creative cognition and brain network dynamics. *Trends in Cognitive Sciences*, 19(8), 434–443. https://doi.org/10.1016/j.tics.2015.05.004

Csikszentmihalyi, M. (1997). *Creativity: Flow and the Psychology of Discovery and Invention* (pp. 67-82). Harper Perennial.

Csikszentmihalyi, M. (1990). Flow: The Psychology of Optimal Experience. Harper & Row.

Fancourt, D., Williamon, A., Carvalho, L. A., Steptoe, A., Dow, R., & Lewis, I. (2016). Singing modulates mood, stress, cortisol, cytokine and neuropeptide activity in cancer patients and carers. *Ecancermedicalscience*, 10, 631. https://doi.org/10.3332/ecancer.2016.631

Gussak D. (2007). The effectiveness of art therapy in reducing depression in prison populations. *International Journal of Offender Therapy Comparative Criminology*,51(4):444-60. doi: 10.1177/0306624X06294137. PMID: 17652148.

Kaufman, J. C., & Beghetto, R. A. (2009). Beyond big and little: The four C model of creativity. *Review of General Psychology, 13*(1), 1–12. https://doi.org/10.1037/a0013688

Kreutz, G., Bongard, S., Rohrmann, S., Hodapp, V., & Grebe, D. (2004). *Effects of choir singing or listening on secretory immunoglobulin A, cortisol, and emotional state. Journal of Behavioral Medicine*, 27(6), 623-635. https://doi.org/10.1007/s10865-004-0006-9

Van Der Kolk, B. (2014). *The Body Keeps the Score: Brain, Mind, and Body in the Healing of Trauma* (pp. 201-220). Penguin Books.

Chapter 9. Self-care Triggers—A Pathway to Mental Wellbeing

Self-care often gets a bad rap, like it's something indulgent or luxurious that you only do when you've got extra time. But here's the reality: selfcare isn't just bubble baths and spa days—it's a vital part of maintaining your mental and emotional health. Think of it as a way to recharge your batteries so you can keep going, especially when life feels overwhelming.

In this chapter, we'll break down what self-care really means, why it's backed by science, and how you can easily integrate it into your everyday life—whether at work, at home, or in between. Spoiler alert: it's not as hard as you think!

The Science Behind Self-care

Self-care might sound simple, but it's actually a powerful way to improve your mental health. Research shows that regular self-care reduces stress, boosts your mood, and helps you cope with anxiety and depression. (Richards, Campenni & Muse-Burke, 2010; Neff, 2011; Riegel et al., 2017; Germer & Neff, 2019)

When we don't take care of ourselves, stress can pile up, leading to problems like burnout, high blood pressure, and even a weakened immune system. It's like never changing the oil in your car—you might keep running for a while, but eventually, things start to break down.

Figure 9.1 is an illustration of a "self-care tool box".

Figure 9.1 The Self-care Toolbox

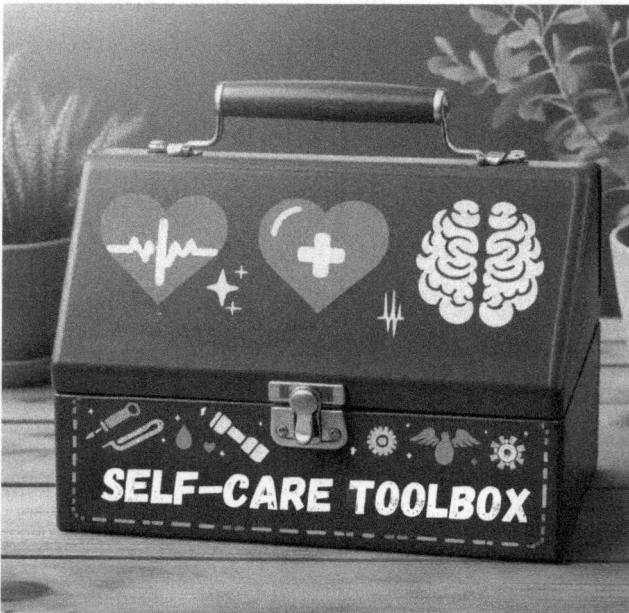

The toolbox concept can be an aid when you encounter situations that require actions to restabilize your sense of balance and position on the issues at hand. I created this image based on my own experience in life when I've had to draw upon my own self-care tools to address or deal with trauma and or life changes. Self-care works by lowering your body's levels of cortisol (the stress hormone) and triggering feel good chemicals like endorphins and dopamine. It doesn't have to be a huge time commitment. Simple actions like getting enough sleep, exercising, or even practicing gratitude can create a positive feedback loop in your brain, making you more resilient to stress and improving your overall mental health.

Why Self-care is So Important for Your Mental Wellbeing

Self-care is more than a wellness buzzword—it's paying attention to daily health-conscious practices to keep your mental and physical health in check. When you make time for selfcare, you're not just pampering yourself, you're boosting your brain chemistry in a way that helps you handle whatever life throws at you. And here's a fun fact: studies have shown that self-care activities like exercise, mindfulness, and creative hobbies can actually reduce symptoms of depression and anxiety.(Pilkington & Wieland, 2020; Marks, February 23, 2024)

So, what's the secret? It's all about balance. Taking care of yourself doesn't mean ignoring your responsibilities; it means making time for small actions that recharge your energy and reset your mind. When you prioritize self-care, you're giving yourself the tools to manage stress and stay grounded.

Practical Self-care Strategies for Work and Home

Here are some self-care triggers—simple, science backed ways to take care of yourself—whether you're at home or on the clock.

1. Positive Affirmation Triggers

Positive affirmations are short, encouraging statements that can help shift your mindset. Studies show that they activate brain regions linked to self-worth and reward, which can improve your mood.

1. *At Home*: Start your day by writing or saying three positive affirmations. For example, "I am enough," "I deserve happiness," or "I can handle whatever comes my way."

2. *At Work*: When stress hits, pause and remind yourself of your strengths. Try a quick mental affirmation like, "I'm capable of doing great work," to re-center yourself.

In fact, Figure 9.2 this point about having positive affirmation triggers.

Figure 9.2. Affirmation Mirror

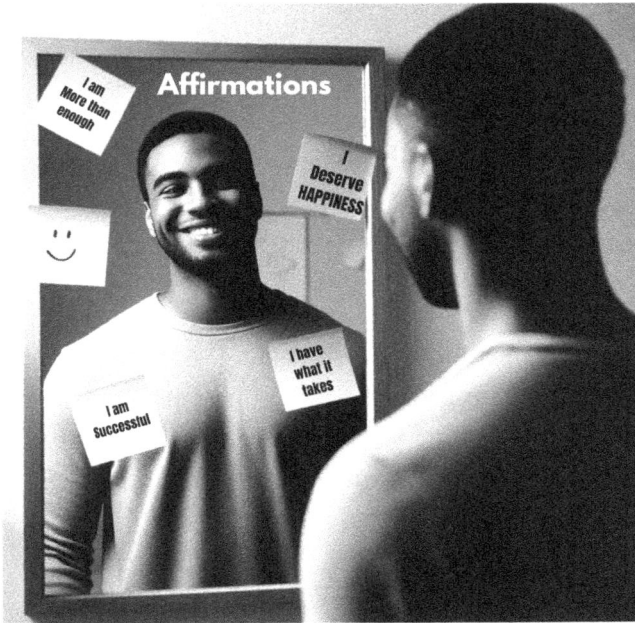

Going through my own life journey, this image highlights the importance of having key affirmation messages that I tell myself daily. It is a practice that can help all of us for maintaining a positive and healthy mindset to balance out the negative triggers we may encounter.

2. Gratitude Triggers

Practicing gratitude has been linked to better mental health, improved mood, and reduced stress. The more you focus on what's good, the easier it becomes to handle life's challenges.

1. *At Home*: Keep a gratitude journal where you write down three things you're thankful for each day. It could be as simple as a sunny day or a good cup of coffee.

2. *At Work*: Start meetings with a positive note, like acknowledging a team achievement or appreciating a colleague's effort. This sets a positive tone and encourages a supportive work environment.

3. Exercise Triggers

Exercise isn't just for your physical health—it's one of the best ways to improve your mental wellbeing. When you move, your body releases endorphins and dopamine, which are natural mood boosters.

1. *At Home*: Aim for 20–30 minutes of activity each day, whether it's a walk, yoga, or dancing in your living room. The key is to move in a way that feels good to you.

2. *At Work*: Take short breaks to stretch or walk around. Even five minutes of movement can shake off stress and refresh your mind.

4. Mindfulness and Meditation Triggers

Mindfulness and meditation are excellent for managing stress and anxiety. Studies show that they can be just as effective as medication in reducing symptoms of anxiety and depression.

1. *At Home*: Dedicate 5–10 minutes a day to mindfulness meditation. Simply focus on your breathing,

and let any wandering thoughts drift by without judgment.

2. *At Work:* Feeling overwhelmed? Take a mindful breathing break. Close your eyes, take a deep breath, and focus on the sensation of breathing. This can instantly calm your mind and reduce tension.

5. Creative Expression Triggers

Creativity is more than just a fun hobby—it's a way to process emotions, reduce anxiety, and boost happiness. Engaging in creative activities helps you enter a "flow state," where time slips away, and you feel deeply engaged in the moment.

1. *At Home:* Try something creative like painting, writing, or playing an instrument. The goal isn't to be perfect—it's to enjoy the process.

2. *At Work*: Tap into your creativity by approaching work tasks from a fresh perspective. Even something as simple as organizing your desk or designing a project outline can be a form of creative expression.

6. Nature Triggers

Spending time outdoors has incredible mental health benefits. Nature helps reduce stress, lower anxiety, and improve your mood. Even just a short walk outside can do wonders.

1. *At Home:* Plan outdoor activities like hiking, gardening, or simply sitting in the park. Nature has a calming effect that helps reset your mind.

2. *At Work:* If possible, take your breaks outside or bring some elements of nature indoors with plants or nature inspired decor.

7. Social Connection Triggers

We're wired for connection. Meaningful relationships are essential for good mental health. Loneliness can increase stress, while positive social interactions release oxytocin, the bonding hormone that makes us feel secure and happy.

1. *At Home:* Make time to connect with friends or family. Even a quick call or text can strengthen relationships and boost your mood.

2. *At Work:* Build rapport with your colleagues. A quick chat or sharing a laugh during the day can ease stress and create a supportive work environment.

8. Self-Compassion Triggers

Being kind to yourself, especially during tough times, is one of the most important forms of self-care. Self-Compassion helps you bounce back from setbacks and reduces feelings of guilt or inadequacy.

1. *At Home:* When you're hard on yourself, take a step back and ask, "What would I say to a friend in this situation?" Treat yourself with that same kindness.

2. *At Work:* Don't let mistakes define you. Instead of criticizing yourself, focus on what you've learned and how you'll move forward.

Building Your Personalized Self-care Routine

To create a self-care routine that works for you, start by identifying the activities that make you feel good. It doesn't have to be complicated—small actions, done consistently, make the biggest impact. Whether it's taking a few minutes each morning for mindfulness or scheduling time for a walk, choose things that fit naturally into your life.

Tracking Your Progress

Staying consistent with self-care is easier when you track your progress. Here are two simple ways to do it:

1. *Daily Self-care Checklist:* Make a list of your self-care activities (e.g., exercise, gratitude, creative expression). Check them off as you go, and give yourself credit for every small step.

2. *Mood Journal:* Record how you feel each day and note how your self-care practices impact your mood. Over time, you'll see which activities have the most positive effect on your wellbeing.

Reflective Exercise

Pause and Evaluate: Take a moment to reflect on how well you prioritize self-care in your daily routine. Consider the following:

- How often do you take intentional breaks to recharge?

- Do you feel emotionally, mentally, or physically drained at the end of the day?

- In what ways are you neglecting your own needs, and how does this impact your mood or energy levels?

- When was the last time you engaged in an activity that nourished your soul or brought you joy?

Action Step: Write down one self-care trigger you can incorporate into your daily routine, whether it's a morning meditation, a 10-minute walk, or calling a friend for support.

Journaling Prompt

Reflect on a time when you felt emotionally or physically drained. What were the circumstances that led to this feeling? What self-care practices could have helped alleviate the stress or burnout? Moving forward, how can you build more consistent self-care habits into your routine?

Conclusion — The Power of Self-care

Self-care isn't selfish—it's essential for your mental health. By making selfcare a priority, you're choosing to invest in your wellbeing and happiness. Whether it's a quick walk, a few minutes of mindfulness, or simply being kind to yourself, these small actions can have a huge impact on how you feel.

In a world that often demands too much of us, self-care is the best way to take back control. It's your time to recharge, reset, and find balance. So go ahead—make selfcare a daily habit and watch how it transforms your life.

Self-care is your key to unlocking resilience, joy, and balance in a hectic world.

Chapter 9 References

Germer, C. K., & Neff, K. D. (2019). *The Mindful Self-Compassion Workbook: A Proven Way to Accept Yourself, Build Inner Strength, and Thrive* (pp. 73-85). The Guilford Press.

Marks, J. L. (2024, February 23). Why self-care can help with depression — plus, 7 science-backed activities to try. *Everyday Health.* Accessed online September 8, 2024 at https://www.everydayhealth.com/depression/why-self-care-can-help-with-depression/

Neff, K. D. (2011). *Self-Compassion: The Proven Power of Being Kind to Yourself* (pp. 50-65). William Morrow.

Pilkington, K., & Wieland, L. S. (2020). Self-care for anxiety and depression: A comparison of evidence from Cochrane reviews and practice to inform decision-making and priority-setting. *BMC Complementary Medicine and Therapies,* 20, 247. https://doi.org/10.1186/s12906-020-03038-8

Riegel, B., Moser, D. K., Buck, H. G., Dickson, V. V., Dunbar, S. B., Lee, C. S., Lennie, T. A., Linderfeld, J., Mitchell J. E., Treat-Jacobson D. J., Webber, D. E., & American Heart Association Council on Cardiovascular and Stroke Nursing; Council on Peripheral Vascular Disease; and Council on Quality of Care and Outcomes Research. (2017). Self-care for the prevention and management of cardiovascular disease and stroke: A scientific statement for healthcare professionals from the American Heart Association. *Journal of the American Heart Association,* 6(9), e006997. DOI: 10.1161/JAHA.117.006997

Richards, K. C., Campenni, C. E., & Muse-Burke, J. L. (2010). Self-care and wellbeing in mental health

professionals: The mediating effects of self-compassion. *Journal of Mental Health Counseling,* 32 (3): 247–264.
https://doi.org/10.17744/mehc.32.3.0n31v88304423806

Chapter 10. Joy in Solitude—Reawakening Your Imagination for Self-Discovery

For much of my life, I thrived in the midst of people. Growing up, I was always the extrovert—the life of the party. As a DJ and party promoter, my world was filled with loud music, packed rooms, and the exhilarating energy of being in the center of it all. I loved it. My weekends were booked with events, and I was constantly interacting with new people, creating unforgettable experiences. It was fun, no doubt, and it helped me build a fan base of people who appreciated my work.

But as I began to shift my focus in life, I realized something crucial: not everyone who gets on your elevator is meant to stay with you for the entire ride. Some people are meant to get off at certain floors. And that's okay.

As I moved away from promoting parties and turned my attention toward personal growth and helping others through mindfulness, I had to leave much of that crowd behind. While I still interact with them and appreciate the relationships I built, my inner circle became smaller—filled with those who aligned with my vision and supported my journey. That's when I began to understand the power of solitude. It wasn't just about who was around me; it was about who I was becoming when I spent time alone.

The Power of Solitude: Rediscovering Your Inner World

When you think about solitude, it often comes with negative connotations. For many people, solitude is synonymous with loneliness or isolation. But there's a difference between loneliness and solitude. Loneliness is the absence of connection, while solitude is the presence of connection—just with yourself. It's in solitude that you can reconnect with your inner world, hear your thoughts without the noise of the outside world, and rediscover the vast landscape of your imagination.

Growing up, I would spend hours in my own world, playing with toys—especially my collection of green army men. I would sit for hours, crafting entire battlefields and creating missions for my toy soldiers. In my solitude, my imagination knew no bounds. The army men weren't just toys; they were part of a greater narrative I built in my mind. They had missions, victories, and challenges. My imagination allowed me to see possibilities beyond my reality, and I created entire worlds from the comfort of my room.

As adults, we often lose touch with that boundless imagination. Life, responsibilities, and expectations tame that creative spark. We become so focused on tasks, to do lists, and external validation that we forget the joy of simply dreaming. But what I've learned through my journey into mindfulness and self-reflection is that solitude isn't about being alone—it's about reawakening that childlike imagination, allowing yourself to dream again, and reimagining where you want to be in life.

It's in the quiet moments, when we step away from the noise of the world, that we have the space to envision the life we want. Solitude gives us permission to imagine that dream job, to visualize the business we've always wanted to start, or to picture ourselves finally writing that book we've put off for years. It's in solitude that we can begin to craft a new mission for ourselves—a mission filled with purpose, fulfillment, and joy.

The Elevator of Life: Knowing When to Let People Off

Life is like an elevator. As we ascend, different people get on at various floors. Some stay with us for a few floors, while others stay longer. But not everyone is meant to ride with us to the top. There comes a point when the elevator gets too crowded, and if you don't have the intuition to recognize when it's time to let some people off, you risk getting stuck—or worse, slowing down your journey.

For me, that realization came when I transitioned from being the life of the party to embracing a more introspective life. I had spent years giving out—giving my energy, my time, and my attention to others. But when I changed my focus and began prioritizing my own growth and purpose, I realized that not everyone could come with me. It wasn't personal. It wasn't about cutting people off; it was about recognizing that we were on different journeys. And if I kept holding on to everyone, my elevator would get stuck or start moving slower.

Solitude is like pressing the pause button on the elevator ride. It's a chance to stop and reflect on who's still with you and who might need to step off. And while it may feel lonely at first, it creates the space for the right people to come into your life—those who align with your vision, purpose, and energy.

My inner circle is now small, but it's filled with people who lift me up, challenge me to be better, and support my mission. That's the power of solitude—it gives you the clarity to know when to let people off your elevator and when to welcome new ones aboard.

Reawakening Your Imagination and Creativity

In solitude, you're not just sitting in silence—you're giving yourself the space to dream again. You're reawakening that imagination that may have been dormant for years. And in doing so, you're planting the seeds for your future.

Think of your thoughts as seeds. You can't get apples from orange seeds, and you can't get bananas from peanut seeds. So why do we think we can reach our goals with negative thoughts, fears, and doubts? Those seeds will only produce more of the same. But when you plant seeds of hope, imagination, and positivity, you begin to attract the life you want.

As a child, I used my imagination to build worlds for my army men. Today, I use my solitude to imagine the world I want to live in—the world where I'm using my gifts to help others, where I'm living in abundance, where I'm living my purpose. Solitude gives you the space to imagine success on your own terms. It allows you to visualize what abundance means to you, whether that's financial wealth, inner peace, or the joy of making a difference in the world.

Imagination isn't just for children—it's a powerful tool for adults, too. And the good news is that it's never too late to reawaken it.

The Science of Solitude: Benefits for Your Mental and Emotional Wellbeing

The benefits of solitude aren't just anecdotal—they're backed by science. Studies have shown that spending time alone can boost creativity, improve emotional regulation, and enhance self-reflection. When we spend time in solitude, our brains process information differently, allowing us to dig deeper into our thoughts and emotions. This leads to greater clarity, better decision making, and a stronger sense of self.

A study published in Personality and Social *Psychology Review* found that people who regularly engage in solitude are better able to regulate their emotions and are less likely to become overwhelmed by stress and anxiety.(Nguyen, 2018) Solitude allows us the time and space to process our emotions in a healthy way, without the distractions of external stimuli. It's a powerful tool for building resilience and emotional strength through increased freedom, creativity and intimacy.(Long & Averill, 2003)

Another study in The *Journal of Personality and Social Psychology* revealed that solitude is linked to increased creativity.(Emmons, & McCullough, 2003) When we're alone, our minds are free to wander, and it's in this mental wandering that new ideas, solutions, and insights often emerge.

Practical Ways to Embrace Solitude

For those of us who are used to being around people, embracing solitude can feel uncomfortable at first. But like any skill, it can be developed over time. Here are a few practical ways to embrace solitude and use it as a tool for self-discovery:

1. *Set Aside Daily Quiet Time:* Start small by setting aside 10-15 minutes of quiet time each day. During this time, practice mindfulness meditation or simply sit in silence. Let your thoughts flow without judgment, and use this time to reconnect with yourself.

This establishes creative boundaries that make space for deep focus, inspiration and creative expression.(Kaufman & Gregoire, 2016)

2. *Use Journaling for Reflection:* Writing is one of the best ways to process emotions and gain clarity. Set aside time each day to journal about your thoughts, feelings, and goals. Use this practice to explore what matters most to you and how you want to shape your life.

3. *Reawaken Your Childhood Creativity:* Just as I once used my green army men to build entire worlds, find a creative activity that allows you to tap into your imagination. Whether it's drawing, writing, or playing music, give yourself the freedom to create without limitations.

4. *Take Solitary Walks in Nature:* Nature is one of the best environments for solitude. Whether you go for a hike or simply sit in a park, nature has a way of calming the mind and giving you space to reflect. Use this time to think about your goals, your dreams, and the life you want to create.

5. *Limit Digital Distractions:* In today's world, solitude is often interrupted by social media and technology. Set boundaries with your devices and take time each day to disconnect.(Gump & Matthews, 1999) Having clear boundaries can prevent distractions, allowing people to fully engage in the present

and reach peak performance.(Csikszentmihalyi, 1990) This will give you the mental space to think deeply and reconnect with your inner self.

Reflective Exercise

Evaluate Your Circle: Take some time to think about the key relationships in your life. Ask yourself:

- Are the people in your life supportive of your growth, or do they drain your energy?

- How do you feel after spending time with certain individuals? Uplifted or exhausted?

- Do your relationships align with your values and emotional needs, or could you be compromising who you are to maintain certain connections?

Action Step: Identify one relationship that enhances your wellbeing and another that may need healthier boundaries. Commit to nurturing the positive relationship and re-evaluating or setting boundaries in the other.

Journaling Prompt

Consider a relationship in your life that is currently causing you stress or tension. What are the underlying issues that contribute to the strain? What steps can you take to address the situation—whether it is through communication, setting boundaries, or letting go? Reflect on how healthier relationships can help positively impact your overall wellbeing.

Conclusion — Embracing the Joy of Solitude

Solitude is not something to be feared—it's a powerful space for growth, creativity, and emotional clarity. By spending intentional time alone, you can reawaken the imagination that once allowed you to dream without limits. You can begin to visualize the life you want, free from the noise and distractions of the outside world.

In solitude, you'll find that true abundance is not just about wealth but about the overflowing fulfillment of every need—where peace, joy, love, and purpose flow as freely as prosperity. Solitude allows you to connect with your inner wisdom and navigate life's challenges with grace and confidence.

Take the time to embrace solitude, reawaken your imagination, and envision the abundant life that's waiting for you.

Chapter 10 References

Csikszentmihalyi, M. (1990). Flow: The Psychology of Optimal Experience. Harper & Row.

Emmons, R. A., & McCullough, M. E. (2003). Counting blessings versus burdens: An experimental investigation of gratitude and subjective well-being in daily life. *Journal of Personality and Social Psychology*, 84(2), 377–389.
https://doi.org/10.1037/0022-3514.84.2.377

Gump, B. B., & Matthews, K. A. (1999). Do background stressors influence reactivity to and recovery from acute stressors? 1. *Journal of Applied Social Psychology*, 29(3), 469-494.
https://doi.org/10.1111/j.1559-1816.1999.tb01397.x

Kaufman, S. B., & Gregoire, C. (2016). Wired to Create: Unraveling the Mysteries of the Creative Mind. Tarcher Perigee.

Long, C. R., & Averill, J. R. (2003). Solitude: An exploration of the benefits of being alone. *Journal of the Theory of Social Behavior*, 33(1), 2144.
https://doi.org/10.1111/1468-5914.00204

Nguyen, T. V., Ryan, R. M., & Deci, E. L. (2018). Solitude as an approach to effective self regulation. *Personality and Social Psychology Review*.
https://doi.org/10.1177/1088868317745914

Chapter 11. The Art of Letting Go—Releasing Control and Embracing Flow

For much of my life, I thrived in the midst of people. Growing up, I was always the extrovert—the life of the party. As a DJ and party promoter, my world was filled with loud music, packed rooms, and the exhilarating energy of being in the center of it all. I loved it. My weekends were booked with events, and I was constantly interacting with new people, creating unforgettable experiences. It was fun, no doubt, and it helped me build a fan base of people who appreciated my work.

But as I began to shift my focus in life, I realized something crucial: not everyone who gets on your elevator is meant to stay with you for the entire ride. Some people are meant to get off at certain floors and that's okay.

There's an old saying that "life is what happens when you're busy making other plans." For a long time, I thought I was the master of those plans, trying to control every detail, every relationship, and every outcome. I believed that if I worked hard enough, gave enough of myself, and helped others grow, everything would fall into place. But what I ended up with was emotional exhaustion, draining relationships, and a deeper understanding of human behavior that I never antici-pated. I was searching for love, but instead, I received an education.

Looking back, I can now see the pattern. I've always had a healing energy—a natural instinct to help and up-lift others. While this is often seen as a positive trait, it became a double-edged sword. Without realizing it, I was attracting people who needed healing—those who were emotionally wounded, broken, and at times manip-ulative. I found myself in relationships with people who had deep abandonment issues, passive aggressive tendencies, and, in some cases, closet narcissism. It was like I had become a magnet for individuals who didn't want to change but expected me to fix them anyway.

I recall a pivotal conversation with my therapist. I was venting about an emotionally exhausting relation-ship where I was dealing with someone who had aban-donment issues, exhibited passive aggressive behavior, and showed narcissistic traits. My therapist paused and said, "Dealing with one of those issues is tough. But dealing with all three? That's a lot." And he was right—it was overwhelming. I found myself constantly walk-ing on eggshells, feeling as though I was somehow re-sponsible for all the emotional turmoil, which eventu-ally drove me into a depressive state.

But through that painful experience, I learned one of the most valuable lessons of my life: the art of letting go. I learned to let go of control, release people who weren't ready to heal, and most importantly, abandon the need for specific outcomes.

When Trauma Becomes the Third Wheel: Recognizing the Patterns

One of the most frustrating parts of being in a relationship with someone who says they want to change is realizing that they may not be ready or willing to do the inner work. I remember telling one of my exes, "It feels like I'm talking to your trauma more than I'm talking to you." In many ways, it was true. Trauma can hijack a person's life, making it difficult for them to see anything beyond their pain.

This realization led me to explore the therapeutic model called Internal Family Systems (IFS).(Brenner, Schwartz, & Becker, 2023; Sweezy, & Ziskind (Eds.), 2013) In IFS, we learn that everyone has different "parts" within themselves, like subpersonalities that emerge to protect them from emotional pain. These parts, such as the "Protector" or the "Firefighter," develop as defense mechanisms to guard against reexperiencing trauma. Ironically, these parts often end up causing more harm than good.

In that relationship, my partner's trauma had created a "Protector" part that continually pushed me away, despite their expressed desire for love and connection. The trauma steered the ship, creating an impenetrable barrier between us. No matter how hard I tried to connect, the wall only grew thicker. It was a bitter pill to swallow, but I realized that I couldn't fix them. They had to do the work themselves, and if they weren't ready, no amount of love or effort from me could change that.

The Power of Letting Go of Control

For someone like me—used to taking charge and fixing problems—letting go of control was one of the hardest things I had to learn. I believed that if I worked hard enough, I could shape the outcome of any situation. But I was wrong. Trying to control everything only led to more suffering and disappointment.

I eventually understood that much of our suffering comes from holding onto expected outcomes. We paint a picture in our minds of how things should go—how relationships should develop, how careers should unfold, how life should be. And when reality doesn't align with these expectations, we experience pain, frustration, and disappointment. The truth is, the more you try to control the outcome, the more you set yourself up for suffering.

This concept became crystal clear to me during one of my most challenging relationships. I clung to the belief that things would get better if I just kept giving. But the more I held onto that expectation, the more miserable I became. When I finally let go—when I accepted that the relationship was what it was and stopped trying to control the outcome—I found peace. Letting go didn't mean giving up; it meant freeing myself from the illusion that I ever had control in the first place.

The Trees Let Go: Lessons from Nature

One of the metaphors that helped me fully embrace letting go came from nature. Trees, in all their wisdom, shed their leaves in the fall without hesitation. They don't try to hold onto those leaves, hoping they'll turn green again. They let them fall because they understand that it's part of the natural cycle. Holding onto dead leaves would only weigh the tree down, preventing it from growing new ones. In the same way, when we hold onto people, situations, or expectations that no longer serve us, we stunt our own growth.

Letting go of control allowed me to see that it wasn't my job to keep people in my life who weren't meant to stay. Some people are like those autumn leaves—they come into our lives for a season, and then it's time to let them go. Holding onto them only weighs us down, and once we release them, we create space for new, healthier experiences to take root.

Releasing the Need to Fix Others

A critical aspect of letting go is releasing the need to fix others. I've always been drawn to people who needed healing, but I had to learn that it's not my responsibility to fix anyone. It's emotionally exhausting and ultimately futile to try to heal someone who isn't ready to heal themselves.

This realization became a kind of superpower for me. After years of emotionally draining relationships, I developed what I call my "Spidey sense." Within 15 to 30 minutes of talking to someone, I could often tell what type of personality I was dealing with. It's almost like a game to me now. I can meet someone and, within moments, describe their personality and insecurities.

However, with that knowledge comes a choice. Just because I can see someone's trauma or wounds doesn't mean it's my job to heal them. The hardest part of this lesson was knowing when to walk away, when to stop trying to fix things, and when to let people go.

Letting Go of Expectations

Another major lesson I learned is the importance of letting go of expected outcomes. So much of our suffering comes from things not going the way we thought they would. We create stories in our minds about how life should unfold, and when reality doesn't match that story, we feel disappointed, hurt, and sometimes even betrayed.

But when you let go of those expectations and allow life to unfold in its own way, you free yourself from constant anxiety and frustration. You stop clinging to what you think should happen and open yourself to the possibility of something even better. Letting go of control and expectations doesn't mean you stop caring; it means you stop forcing things to go your way. It's about embracing the flow of life and trusting that things will happen as they are meant to.

Practical Tools for Letting Go

If you struggle with control like I did, here are some practical steps to help you let go:

1. Identify Your Control Triggers

Notice the areas where you feel the most need for control. Is it in your relationships, career, or family dynamics? Once you identify these areas, ask yourself why you feel the need to control them. What fear is driving this behavior? Understanding the root cause is the first step in letting go.

2. Practice Mindfulness

Mindfulness helps you stay present and accept things as they are rather than constantly trying to change them. When you feel the need to control a situation, pause and ask yourself, "Is this something I can control?" If the answer is no, let it go.

3. Release Expectations

A major part of letting go is releasing your expectations of how things should be. Practice accepting what is, rather than what you think should be.

4. Set Boundaries

Letting go doesn't mean allowing people to walk all over you. Setting healthy boundaries is crucial. Know when to say no, when to step back, and when to protect your energy. You can't control others, but you can control how much access they have to you.

In fact, Figure 11.1 is a simple illustration based on my own reflection of the importance of visualizing healthy boundaries.

Figure 11.1 Visualizing Healthy Boundaries

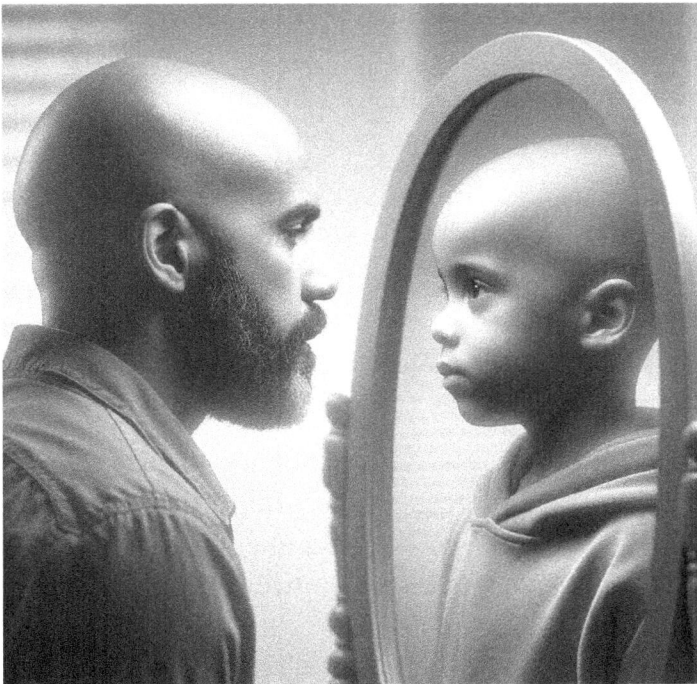

This illustration highlights the importance of connecting with and understanding my inner child as a foundation for setting boundaries in life. We can learn from the healing needed from childhood wounds to protect and strengthen our emotional space for ourselves as adults. This also better enables us to be helpful and supportive of others.

The Gift of Letting Go

Letting go has been one of the hardest lessons for me, but also one of the most liberating. The relationships that once drained me, the need to control every situation, the expectations that weighed me down—I've learned to release them. And in doing so, I've created space for peace, joy, and abundance in my life.

Abundance isn't just about material wealth. As I often say, "Abundance is more than wealth; it's the overflowing fulfillment of every need—where peace, joy, love, and purpose flow as freely as prosperity. True abundance is when your heart and soul feel just as rich as your pockets."

Letting go allows that abundance to flow into your life in the form of peace, love, and fulfillment. So, take a deep breath, release the need to control, and trust that life will unfold in its own beautiful way.

Reflective Exercise

Take a moment to reflect on a situation, relationship, or past experience that you've been holding on to—something that has weighed on your mind or heart for a long time. Close your eyes, and take a few deep breaths. Visualize yourself standing on a hilltop, with the weight of that situation in a backpack on your shoulders. With each breath, feel the weight of it. Now, imagine slowly removing the backpack, and watch it roll down the hill, disappearing into the distance.

Once you feel that burden leaving you, ask yourself the following:

How do I feel now that I've let go of this weight?

What emotions arise when I imagine freeing myself from this?

How might letting go of this situation or burden change my daily life?

Journaling Prompt

Write about something you've been holding onto, whether it's a relationship, a grudge, or a past mistake. Why do you think it's been hard for you to let it go?

Now imagine what your life would look like if you no longer carried that burden. How would it change your perspective, your mood, or your actions?

What steps can you take, starting today, to actively release this and move forward?

Write freely, allowing yourself to express your thoughts and emotions. Don't worry about structure—just let the words flow and see what insights come up as you explore the art of letting go in your own life.

Conclusion

Letting go is not about forgetting the past or dismissing the challenges we've faced. Instead, it's about freeing ourselves from the emotional weight that holds us back, allowing space for growth, healing, and new opportunities. By releasing the grip of resentment, pain, and fear, we invite peace and clarity into our lives. Letting go is an art—an ongoing practice that helps us cultivate resilience and embrace the present with a lighter heart. As you move forward, remember that letting go is not a one-time event but a continuous journey. It's about choosing freedom over attachment, joy over bitterness, and peace over conflict.

As you deepen your practice of letting go, you'll discover a profound sense of liberation and a renewed ability to embrace life's challenges with grace and strength. The art of letting go allows you to reclaim your power, align with your true self, and create a future unburdened by the past. It's not just an act of release—it's an invitation to live more fully, authentically, and joyfully.

Chapter 11 References

Brenner, E. G., Schwartz, R. C., & Becker, C. (2023). Development of the internal family systems model: Honoring contributions from family systems therapies. *Family process*, 62(4), 1290-1306. https://doi.org/10.1111/famp.12943

Sweezy, M., & Ziskind, E. L. (Eds.). (2013). Internal family systems therapy: New dimensions. Routledge.

Chapter 12. Digital Detox Triggers – Reclaiming Your Mind in a Hyperconnected World

In today's world, we are more connected than ever before. Notifications, messages, emails, social media updates—all are at our fingertips 24/7. But while our devices promise connection, they often deliver the opposite. Instead of fostering meaningful interactions, technology may leave people of all ages feeling drained, distracted, and anxious.(Gazzaley & Rosen, 2016; Twenge, 2017) This is where the need for a digital detox arises— a much needed break from the constant barrage of information that overwhelms our minds.

One of the most eye-opening moments I had with a client involved reviewing how they were spending their time. They were stressed, disconnected, and constantly behind on their goals. When I asked them about their daily routine, they confessed to spending two hours a day on social media—scrolling, liking, and watching videos. Initially, that didn't seem like much, but when we added it up over the course of a year, the total was staggering: 730 hours, or nearly 30 full days spent on social media alone.

Imagine what could be accomplished with that time. In 730 hours, you could have read 20-30 books, written the first draft of a novel, learned a new language, completed an online course, or even started a side business. You could have deepened your relationships, reconnected with yourself, or simply rested and recharged. The issue isn't about demonizing technology—it's about recognizing the need for balance. Our time and energy are increasingly drained by the digital world, and it's essential to reclaim control.

The Hidden Costs of Being Hyperconnected

Many people are surprised when they realize just how much their devices affect their mental health. Studies show that excessive social media use is directly correlated with increased anxiety, depression, and loneliness.(Andreassen, Pallesen, & Griffiths, 2017; Hunt et al., 2018; Przybylski & Weinstein, 2017; Kross et al., 2013)

Constantly comparing our lives to others' highlight reels, being inundated with negative news, and enduring endless notifications create a cycle of stress and distraction that prevents us from living fully in the present. Figure 12.1 illustrates this point as it can be more difficult to try and keep up with what everyone around us is doing rather than just letting go.

Figure 12.1 Control Balloon

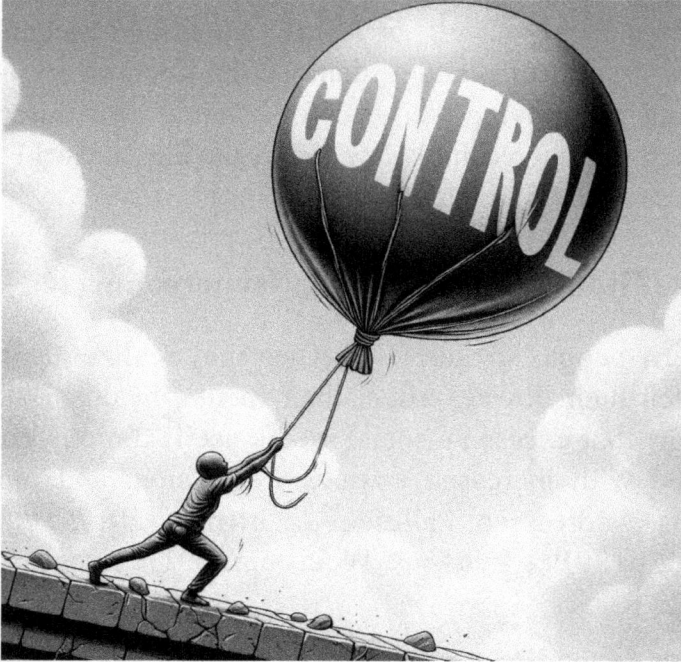

The balloon symbolizes the 'lift' that we can feel and the increased anxiety and stress in these situations. This is compared to when we just release from the comparisons to others and focus on what is good in our own life and what is within our span of control.

It's like eating junk food every day, it might feel good at first, but over time, it takes a serious toll on your body and mind. Similarly, when we consume surface level content, negative news, or endless comparisons on social media, our mental "diet" becomes toxic. We lose focus, our energy drops, and our creativity fades.

Digital Inputs: Protecting Your Mental Space

A key lesson I've learned personally and in my coaching work is the importance of protecting your inputs. Just as we need to be mindful of what we put into our bodies, we must also be vigilant about what we allow into our minds. The energy you consume through social media, news, and the people around you shapes your thoughts, actions, and ultimately, your life.

If your social media feed is filled with negativity, drama, or meaningless content, that's the energy you're absorbing, and that's the energy you're carrying throughout your day. It's no surprise if you feel anxious, drained, or uninspired.

I once had a client who felt stuck, constantly comparing themselves to others on social media. They didn't understand why they always felt inadequate. After a closer look at their feed, we discovered it was full of influencers showcasing their "perfect" lives—flawless bodies, six figure businesses, luxurious vacations. My client was spending two hours a day comparing themselves to an unrealistic version of reality.

We decided to take action. They began unfollowing accounts that didn't serve them and replaced them with content that inspired personal growth, positivity, and balance. The result was almost immediate. Within weeks, they reported feeling more confident, motivated, and energized, and began pursuing their own goals without the constant pressure of comparison.

The Power of a Digital Detox

A digital detox isn't about cutting yourself off from technology entirely. It's about resetting your relationship with your devices and reclaiming your mental space.(Cabrera & Lee, 2020) It's about stepping away from the noise, so you can reconnect with what truly matters—yourself, your goals, your relationships. Figure 12.2 symbolizes the digital inputs impacting us and how a digital detox can help.

Figure 12.2 How a Digital Detox Helps

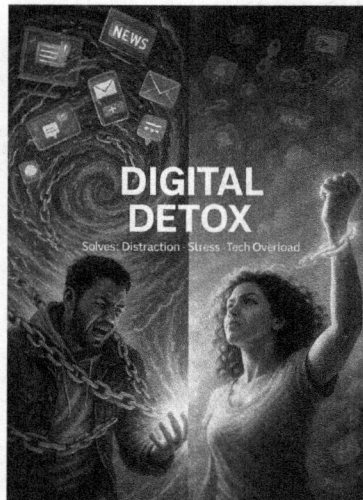

Think of it like taking a vacation to rest and recharge. But how often do we give our minds the same break from the constant barrage of digital stimuli?

I often challenge my clients to try a digital detox for just one week. The results are always eye opening. They feel more focused, more present, and more in tune with their emotions. The anxiety that once felt ever present begins to fade, replaced by a sense of calm and clarity.

One of the biggest benefits of a digital detox is the time you regain. Take the client who was spending two hours a day on social media. By reducing that time by just half to one hour per day, they would free up 365 hours in a year. That's over 15 full days of time that could be redirected toward more meaningful pursuits.

Imagine what you could do with an extra 365 hours. You could:

1. Read 10-15 books,

2. Master a new skill or hobby,

3. Spend quality time with family and friends,

4. Complete a certification course or online class, or

5. Start a side business or creative project.

The possibilities are endless when you reclaim your time and energy.

Practical Steps for a Digital Detox

If you're ready to reclaim your mind and your time, here are some practical steps to help you start a digital detox and protect your mental space:

1. Start Small: Set Time Limits

You don't need to go cold turkey. Start by setting small, achievable goals, like limiting your social media use to 30 minutes per day. Most smartphones have built in screen time trackers that can help you set boundaries.

2. Create "TechFree" Zones

Designate certain areas of your home as techfree zones. For example, make your bedroom a sanctuary for rest by keeping your phone out of reach.(Zaidi et al., 2024) This simple change can improve your sleep and help you wind down at the end of the day.

3. Replace Screen Time with Meaningful Activities

When you reduce screen time, fill that newfound space with activities that enrich your life. Spend time outdoors, engage in creative projects, read books that inspire you, or take up a new hobby. This will not only help you reclaim your time but also nourish your mental and emotional wellbeing.

4. Do a Social Media Audit

Take a critical look at your social media feeds. Unfollow accounts that bring negativity, comparison, or stress into your life. Replace them with content that uplifts, educates, or aligns with your goals. Remember, you control what you consume.

5. Set Boundaries with Technology

Just as you would with people, set clear boundaries with your devices. Turn off notifications that constantly pull you back into the digital world. Set specific times during the day to check emails or social media, and stick to those windows. Evidence has proven that there is a definite need for these boundaries to prevent fatigue and impacts on our mental wellness. (Lee, Son & Kim, 2016)

Real World Connection: Balancing Online and Offline Life

One of the most important benefits of a digital detox is how it helps foster real world connections. It's easy to mistake social media interactions for meaningful relationships, but nothing replaces face to face interaction or genuine conversations. When you step away from your screen, you create space for deeper, more meaningful relationships with the people around you.

I encourage my clients to schedule more in person meetups with friends or family, take walks without their phones, and engage in hobbies that don't involve a screen. These small changes can have a profound impact on happiness and wellbeing.

You Can Stay Informed Without Being Consumed

One of the biggest concerns people have about reducing screen time is staying informed. We live in a world where news is constant, and there's a fear of missing out on important updates. But the truth is, you can stay informed without being consumed.

It's all about balance. You don't need to check the news every hour or stay updated on every trending topic. Choose a reliable news source and set aside time once or twice a day to catch up on headlines. This way, you stay informed without being overwhelmed by constant updates.

Reflective Exercise

1. *Set a Timer:* For the next 24 hours, set a timer each time you pick up your phone, scroll through social media, or spend time on other digital devices. At the end of the day, look at how much time you've spent connected digitally. Reflect on how this impacted your mood, focus, and productivity.

2. *Create a Mindfulness Break:* Set aside 30 minutes to an hour to disconnect from all devices. During this time, practice mindfulness by being fully present in whatever you choose to do—whether it's a walk-in nature, reading a book, journaling, or simply sitting quietly. Afterward, reflect on how this digital break made you feel. Did you experience any challenges, or did it feel like a relief to step away from the screen?

Incorporate this mindfulness break into your routine and notice how small periods of disconnection can enhance your mental clarity and overall sense of well-being.

Journaling Prompt

> How has constant connectivity impacted your mental and emotional health? Write about times when you've felt overwhelmed by digital interactions. What strategies can you implement to create healthier boundaries with technology moving forward?

Conclusion — Reclaiming Your Mind

The digital world is here to stay, and it offers many benefits. But when we let it dominate our lives, it drains our energy, distracts us from our goals, and leaves us feeling disconnected. A digital detox is about reclaiming control—protecting your mental space and making room for the things that truly matter.

Remember, your time is valuable. Don't let it slip away through endless scrolling, comparison, or distraction. By reclaiming your time and protecting your inputs, you can cultivate a life filled with focus, connection, and joy.

Chapter 12 References

Andreassen, CS, Pallesen S, & Griffiths MD. (2017). The relationship between addictive use of social media, narcissism, and self esteem: Findings from a large national survey. *Addictive Behaviors*, 64, 287293. https://doi.org/10.1016/j.addbeh.2016.03.006

Cabrera JF, & Lee R. (2020). The influence of a digital detox intervention on wellbeing. *Cyberpsychology, Behavior, and Social Networking*, 23(9), 619625. https://doi.org/10.1089/cyber.2019.0803

Gazzaley, A., & Rosen, L. D. (2016). The distracted mind: Ancient brains in a high-tech world. MIT Press.

Hunt MG, Marx R, Lipson C, & Young J. (2018). No more FOMO: Limiting social media decreases loneliness and depression. *Journal of Social and Clinical Psychology*, 37(10), 751768. https://doi.org/10.1521/jscp.2018.37.10.751

Kross, E, Verduyn, P., Demiralp, E., Park, J., Lee, D. S., Lin, N., Shablack H, Jonides J, & Ybarra, O. (2013). Facebook use predicts declines in subjective wellbeing in young adults. *PLoS ONE*, 8(8), e69841. https://doi.org/10.1371/journal.pone.0069841

Lee AR, Son SM, & Kim KK. (2016). Information and communication technology overload and social networking service fatigue: A stress perspective. *Computers in human behavior*, *55*, 51-61. http://dx.doi.org/10.1016/j.chb.2015.08.011

Przybylski AK, & Weinstein N. (2017). A large scale test of the Goldilocks Hypothesis: Quantifying the relations between digital screen use and the mental wellbeing of adolescents. *Psychological Science*, 28(2), 204215.

https://doi.org/10.1177/0956797616678438

Twenge JM. (2017). iGen: Why Today's SuperConnected Kids Are Growing Up Less Rebellious, More Tolerant, Less Happy And Completely Unprepared for Adulthood. Atria Paperback.

Zaidi, H., AlJadaan, O. T., Al Faress, M. Y., & Jabas, A. O. (2024). Disconnect to Reconnect: Your Path to Physical and Mental Wellbeing. In Exploring Youth Studies in the Age of AI (pp. 25-43). IGI Global.

Chapter 13. Play, Laughing and Singing Triggers – Reclaiming the Joy of Childlike Fun

Life can sometimes feel like a never-ending series of obligations, deadlines, and responsibilities. But amidst the hustle, we often forget the simple joy of play, laughter, and singing—the things that used to make us feel alive as children. We remember what it was like to laugh so hard we cried, to play without any rules or deadlines, and to sing, even if we couldn't carry a tune. That childlike joy is still within us, waiting to be reawakened.

Growing up, I was the life of the party, always surrounded by music, laughter, and fun. Even today, I'm known for my lip-syncing videos on social media that somehow garner half a million views, despite the fact that I'm not a singer. People aren't drawn to my musical talent—they're drawn to the fun, energy, and pure joy I bring to the performance. That's what this chapter is about—reclaiming that joy, regardless of talent or skill, and allowing ourselves to play, laugh, and sing without inhibition.

The Science Behind Play, Laughter and Singing

You might think that laughter, play, and singing are just distractions, but there's real science behind their benefits. Engaging in these activities releases feel good hormones like endorphins and dopamine while reducing cortisol, the hormone responsible for stress.(Fredrickson, 2001; Lester, & Russell, 2010) In other words, when we allow ourselves to laugh, play, and sing, we're giving our brains a natural boost, improving both our mental and physical health.

Laughter, in particular, has been shown to lower blood pressure, reduce tension, and even boost the immune system. It's a powerful tool for stress relief and emotional connection through humor.(Fry, 1994) When you laugh with others, you bond through shared joy, creating a sense of community and support.

Singing, even if you're not a skilled vocalist, offers similar benefits. It improves lung capacity, reduces anxiety, and increases oxytocin, the hormone responsible for feelings of connection and trust. Whether you're singing alone or with others, the physical act of vocalizing can lift your spirits and reduce stress.

Singing Triggers: Healing Through Song (Even If You Can't Sing)

Singing has always been a passion of mine, even though I know I'm not winning any talent shows. But here's the thing—it doesn't matter. What matters is the joy that comes from letting go and singing your heart out. Science backs this up: singing reduces stress, increases feelings of happiness, and strengthens connections with others, even if you're off key.(Gick, 2011)

Why Singing Works:

1. *Endorphins and oxytocin:* These chemicals are released when we sing, helping to reduce stress, improve mood, and create bonds with others.

2. *Reduced anxiety:* Studies show that singing lowers cortisol, the hormone responsible for stress.

3. *Boosts confidence:* It takes bravery to sing, especially when you're not a professional. But every time you let yourself sing, you build confidence and let go of the fear of judgment.

In my own life, I've seen the impact that singing—even badly—can have. My lip-syncing videos may not showcase a golden voice, but they showcase joy, and that's what people connect with. The fun and energy I put into those performances come back to me tenfold through the laughter and positivity they generate. And that's a happiness trigger we can all tap into.

Laughter: The Ultimate Stress Reliever

Laughter is a universal language that lightens even the heaviest of moments. I've always loved comedy, and I use it in my life to tackle serious topics—from aging to health challenges. The ability to laugh at life's hardships, to find humor in the struggles, opens the door to healing. Laughter creates space for difficult conversations, reduces tension, and fosters a sense of connection.(Berk et al., 1989; Provine, 2001)

Benefits of Laughter:

1. *Boosts the immune system:* Laughing increases the production of antibodies, strengthening the body's defenses against illness.

2. *Natural pain relief:* Endorphins released during laughter act as the body's natural painkillers.

3. *Improved mood:* Laughter reduces stress hormones like cortisol, making it easier to manage anxiety and depression.

Incorporating laughter into your daily life is one of the easiest and most effective ways to improve your wellbeing. Whether through a comedy show, a funny podcast, or just calling up a friend who always makes you laugh, you're giving yourself a natural remedy for stress.

Play: Rediscovering Childlike Fun

As adults, we often forget to play. But play is not just for children—it's an essential part of maintaining emotional health. Play stimulates creativity, relieves stress, and brings us into the present moment. It's a form of expression that allows us to explore without the pressure of results.

How to Incorporate Play into Your Life:

1. *Be spontaneous:* Let yourself engage in activities for the sheer joy of it, without an agenda or goal. Whether it's a game, a dance, or a playful conversation, the act of play helps break the monotony of adult responsibilities.

2. *Indulge in creative hobbies:* Whether it's drawing, building, or storytelling, play allows you to tap into your imagination and creativity. The key is to let go of the need for perfection and just enjoy the process.

For me, it was my toy soldiers as a child that unlocked hours of play, and as an adult, I still find ways to engage that sense of wonder. Play doesn't just relieve stress; it reconnects us with our creative selves, reminding us of the joy that comes from simply letting go.

The Energy You Put Out Comes Back to You

One of the greatest lessons I've learned is that the energy you put out into the world comes back to you. When you bring joy, laughter, and kindness to others, that same energy reflects back into your life. Whether it's through singing, laughing, or playing, the joy you spread will find its way back to you.

Practical Ways to Spread Joy:

1. *Share your talent:* Whether it's singing, telling jokes, or playing music, find ways to share your joy with others. Perform in a public space, post

something fun on social media, or just brighten a friend's day.

2. *Be a source of laughter:* Make it your mission to make someone laugh every day. Share a joke, send a funny meme, or call a friend just to spread some humor.

3. *Create a joyful environment:* Fill your space with things that make you smile. Whether it's a playlist of your favorite songs, a comedy podcast, or photos of good memories, surrounding yourself with joy will have a lasting impact on your mood.

Reflective Exercise

Spend 10 minutes in a quiet, comfortable space. Close your eyes and visualize the person or situation that has caused you pain. Imagine the weight of that burden lifting from your shoulders. As you exhale, release the negative emotions you've been holding onto. Reflect on how it feels to let go and make room for healing. Afterward, write down your feelings and any insights you gained during this exercise.

Journaling Prompt

Think about a situation or person in your life where forgiveness has been challenging. How has holding onto resentment or anger affect your emotional, mental, or physical health? What would change if you allowed yourself to forgive? Write about what steps you could take toward forgiveness and how you imagine it might bring healing.

Conclusion — Joy Is Contagious—Spread It

Life doesn't have to be so serious all the time. By tapping into the power of play, laughter, and singing, we can reclaim the joy that often gets buried under the weight of adult responsibilities. These Happiness Triggers aren't just for children—they're essential tools for living a balanced, joyful life.

So, sing out loud, laugh often, and play like you did when you were a kid. The energy you put out is the energy you'll get back, so why not make it joy?

Chapter 13 References

Berk, L. S., Tan, S. A., Fry, W. F., Napier, B. J., Lee, J. W., Hubbard, R. W., ... & Eby, W. C. (1989). Neuroendocrine and stress hormone changes during mirthful laughter. The American journal of the medical sciences, 298(6), 390-396. DOI: 10.1097/00000441-198912000-00006

Fredrickson, B. L. (2001). The role of positive emotions in positive psychology: The broaden-and-build theory of positive emotions. *American Psychologist, 56*(3), 218-226. https://doi.org/10.1037/0003-066X.56.3.218

Fry, W. F. (1994). The biology of humor. Humor: International *Journal of Humor Research.* https://doi.org/10.1515/humr.1994.7.2.111

Gick, M. L. (2011). Singing, health and well-being: A health psychologist's review. *Psychomusicology: Music, Mind and Brain, 21*(1-2), 176–207. https://doi.org/10.1037/h0094011.

Provine, R. R. (2001). Laughter: A Scientific Investigation. Penguin Books.

Lester, S. & Russell, W. (2010). Children's right to play: An examination of the importance of play in the lives of children worldwide. Working Paper No. 57. The Hague, The Netherlands: Bernard van Leer Foundation.

Chapter 14. Happiness Triggers 101: A Guide for Mentors, Parents and Teachers

Let's face it: mental health conversations can feel intimidating, especially if you didn't grow up discussing these topics yourself. Studies, like one from Tampa Bay Thrives, show that many parents and mentors feel ill-equipped to talk about mental health. But here's the good news—you don't need a psychology degree to make a positive impact. You just need a bit of guidance, a sprinkle of courage, and a handful of Happiness Triggers.

This chapter is designed to help you feel more comfortable and confident in fostering mental health conversations, guiding young people to embrace resilience, gratitude, and self-awareness. Think of this as a toolkit to unlock the mental and emotional well-being superpowers we all carry—and yes, there's humor and encouragement along the way.

Why Happiness Triggers are Essential for Emotional Health

In a world filled with endless challenges, equipping young people with Happiness Triggers can make all the difference. Happiness Triggers, in essence, are proactive tools—acts, habits, and mindsets that build mental resilience. They don't erase challenges, but they do help young people manage and respond to them with grace and grit. Research shows that incorporating positive mental habits like gratitude, mindfulness, and self-compassion can reshape how we handle stress, process emotions, and build connections.(Fredrickson, 2001; Emmons & McCullough, 2003)

Building Mental Health Conversations into Everyday Life

Let's make this less intimidating: mental health doesn't need to be a "serious talk" topic. The more you weave it into daily conversations, the more natural and approachable it becomes. Below are some strategies and scenarios to help you seamlessly introduce mental health topics, without feeling like you need a therapy couch and a clipboard.

1. Create a Safe Space for Open Conversations

Young people are more likely to open up if they feel safe and understood. Start with an environment that's free of judgment. Try sharing a small personal story first; this shows that vulnerability is okay and makes the other person feel more comfortable.

Practice Scenario:

Let's say you want to encourage a young person to open up about their day. You could say:

"I had a pretty challenging day, and talking about it really helps me. Is there anything on your mind you'd like to share? No pressure—just know I'm here."

2. Introduce the Concept of 'Thought Triggers'

One way to make the topic of mental health less overwhelming is by discussing "Thought Triggers" instead of directly diving into "mental health." For example, you can explain how certain thoughts can trigger different feelings, like happiness or worry.

Try This:

"I've noticed that certain things make me feel really happy, like taking a walk or reading a good book. Do you have any activities that make you feel good?"

By focusing on activities that positively affect mood, you're gently introducing mental health without diving too deep too fast. This also helps young people develop self-awareness about their own emotional responses.

3. Introduce Mindfulness Through Simple Practices

Mindfulness can sound intimidating, but it doesn't have to be. You can introduce mindfulness as simply "being present" or "paying attention to the moment." Even short activities, like breathing exercises or "mindful listening," can be powerful in grounding young people.

Practice Scenario:

"Want to try something? Let's take five deep breaths together, focusing only on our breathing. This helps me calm down, especially on busy days. Give it a shot?"

Pro Tip:

Kids love hands-on activities, so turn mindfulness into a game. Ask them to notice five things they see, hear, or feel around them. This can help center them in a fun, engaging way.

4. Discuss Feelings as Colors or Weather

Sometimes, talking about emotions in abstract terms—like colors or weather—makes it easier to share without fear. Encourage kids to describe their feelings as a color, or ask, "If your feelings were the weather today, what would it be?" This gives them a framework for expression that doesn't feel as intense.

Practice Scenario:

After a rough day, you could say:

"If you had to choose a color to describe how you're feeling, what would it be?" or "If your mood were the weather, would it be sunny, cloudy, or stormy?"

5. Affirm Their Experiences and Feelings

Acknowledge their feelings as valid, even if they're having a tough time. Avoid jumping to "fix it" mode—sometimes, the best support is simply saying, "I understand, and it's okay to feel this way." This approach not only validates their emotions but also teaches empathy and self-compassion.

Try This

"It sounds like you're feeling pretty frustrated, and that's okay. Everyone has days like that. You can talk to me anytime."

Reflective Exercise: Practice Scenarios with a Peer

Before diving into these conversations, consider practicing with another adult. Practicing scenarios with a friend or partner can help you feel more comfortable with your approach. Here are a few example scenarios:

1. *Discussing a Challenging Day:* Practice how you'd respond if a child shares a tough experience. How would you acknowledge their feelings without rushing to fix them?

2. *Encouraging Gratitude:* Try ways to gently guide gratitude without it feeling forced. Maybe practice phrasing like, "What's something today that you enjoyed, no matter how small?"

3. *Helping Them Calm Down:* Practice introducing a breathing exercise or mindfulness game to help a young person process frustration or anxiety.

Journaling Prompt

> Reflecting on your own comfort with mental health, take a few minutes to reflect on your comfort level with mental health topics. Write down any reservations or fears you might have, and ask yourself why they exist. Are they rooted in your own experiences?

Next, answer these questions:

- What are my goals for having these conversations?
- What's one thing I can do to make these conversations feel more natural?

Conclusion — Growing Together, One Happiness Trigger at a Time

Remember, you're not expected to be perfect or to have all the answers. The fact that you're willing to have these conversations—no matter how uncomfortable or awkward they might feel at first—means you're giving young people a tremendous gift. You're modeling openness, vulnerability, and resilience. These are all Happiness Triggers in action.

And as you go along, remember that this journey is a shared one. Just as much as you're teaching them, you're learning, too. There's beauty in being a lifelong student of life, exploring happiness, resilience, and connection. With each conversation, you're building an emotional toolkit that you can both carry for life.

Let's keep sharing, learning, and making room for happiness in ways big and small. Here's to more sunny days, more calming breaths, and the confidence to be exactly who you—and those you mentor—are meant to be.

Chapter 14 References

Emmons, R. A., & McCullough, M. E. (2003). Counting blessings versus burdens: An experimental investigation of gratitude and subjective well-being in daily life. *Journal of Personality and Social Psychology*, 84(2), 377–389. https://doi.org/10.1037/0022-3514.84.2.377

Fredrickson, B. L. (2001). The role of positive emotions in positive psychology: The broaden-and-build theory of positive emotions. *American Psychologist*, 56(3), 218–226. https://doi.org/10.1037/0003-066X.56.3.218

Schlegel, R. J., Hicks, J. A., Arndt, J., & King, L. A. (2017). The paradoxical link between authenticity and well-being: Authenticity fosters well-being but conceals its trajectory. *Social Psychological and Personality Science*, 8(2), 201–209.
https://doi.org/10.1177/1948550616661016

Chapter 15. Happiness Triggers for Survivors of Domestic Violence

Opening Story and Perspective

I will never forget working on an episode of *Law & Order: SVU* where the storyline centered on a male survivor of sexual assault harmed not by a stranger, but by his parole officer. The room went quiet because it challenged a myth many still hold: abuse has one look, one gender, one story. It doesn't. Domestic violence and coercion can touch anyone, women, men, LGBTQ+ people across every income, culture, and neighborhood.

Data from the National Domestic Violence Hotline shows that most female victims of intimate partner violence are re-victimized by the same offender—77% for women aged 18 to 24, and 76% for women aged 25 to 34. This underscores the dangerous cycle of abuse, where recurrence is highly likely and often escalates in severity.(National Domestic

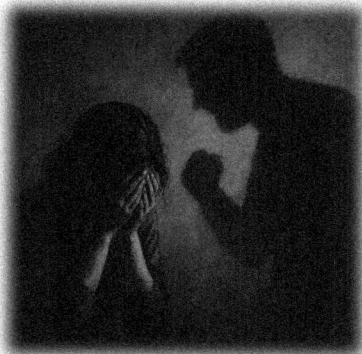

Violence Hotline, ND; World Health Organization, 2021; Basile, et al., 2022)

As a former Board of Directors member with the National Association of Mental Illness (NAMI) in Hillsborough County, FL, I've watched survivors reclaim their lives when they had a plan, support and practical tools. This chapter is a plain-language manual: what abuse is, how to spot its patterns, how to build a safe exit, and how to retrain your mind toward safety and joy with simple, repeatable *Happiness Triggers*.

Understanding Domestic Violence Beyond the Stereotypes

Domestic violence is not just bruises. It's a **pattern of power and control**. That pattern can be physical (hitting, choking, blocking doorways), sexual (any act without consent, reproductive coercion), emotional/psychological (insults, humiliation, threats, isolation), financial (controlling money, sabotaging work, debt in your name), or digital (location tracking, spyware, smart-home intimidation). The common thread isn't "anger" it's **control**.(CDC May 16, 2024; Mulligan 2009; Kelly & Johnson 2008)

Stereotypes keep people silent. Survivors often minimize what's happening because "it's not that bad" or "they never hit me." But the absence of bruises doesn't mean the absence of abuse. If you are being isolated, threatened, humiliated, controlled, or coerced, that is abuse. Naming it does not make you disloyal; it makes

159

you safe.(Seelau & Seelau 2005; Esqueda & Harrison 2005)

It helps to shift the question from "Is it bad enough to leave?" to "Is it safe enough to stay?" That one shift can give you permission to protect yourself sooner.

Recognizing the Early Warning Signs

Abuse usually starts quietly: checking your phone "for your safety," needing your passwords "to be transparent," turning jokes into put-downs, "testing" your loyalty by asking you to cancel plans, or making your money "our" money while limiting your access. One sign becomes three; your world gets smaller.

Common red flags include escalating jealousy, repeated accusations, rage over small things, rules about what you wear or who you see, and **gaslighting**, denying obvious events or telling you you're "too sensitive" or "crazy."(Tsopp-Pagan 2024; Kearney & O'Brien 2021; Women, et al., 1992) If you're walking on eggshells most days, your body already knows you're not safe.

Write a single sentence that names the pattern you see: "They control my (**time/money/phone/friends**) by (**specific example**)." Clarity is step one.

The First Time It Happens: Why It's Critical to Act

Preparation isn't dramatic; it's thoughtful. You can love someone and still refuse to be harmed. You can hope for change and still plan for safety. If the best never happens, you've lost nothing by preparing. If the worst comes, you've already built your lifeboat.

Start with three moves in the next 48 hours: copy key documents to a safe place, identify one trusted person, and look up your local hotline to explore options confidentially.

Building an Exit Strategy

An exit plan is more than "just leave." It's where you'll go, how you'll get there, what you'll bring, and who will help, is it timed for the safest window. Connect with your local domestic violence hotline to create a **personalized safety plan**; advocates do this every day and can suggest details you might miss.(Sabri, et al., 2022; Murray, et al., 20215)

Core steps: stash small amounts of cash; photograph IDs, birth certificates, insurance cards, bank info, and court orders and upload to a secure cloud; pack a discreet "go bag" (meds, keys, prepaid phone, charger, clothes, copies of documents, pet records); create a code word with a friend ("Check the recipe" = call 911); choose two safe locations (a friend, a shelter) and two routes to each. If police respond, ask whether they use a

lethality assessment and request an advocate handoff.(Grant & Cross-Denny, 2024; Klein 2012)

Leaving can be the most dangerous time; this is why stealth, timing, and support matter. Plan slow on paper so you can move fast if needed.

Financial Abuse and Digital Control

Money and tech are modern tethers. Financial abuse shows up as forced "allowances," blocking you from work, taking your paychecks, or opening credit in your name. Digital abuse uses shared Apple IDs, hidden AirTags, spyware, or smart-home devices to monitor or intimidate. If your devices feel unsafe, assume they might be.

Open a private account if you can (credit union accounts can be easier); start a small "freedom fund" even with coins; keep a photo of your documents stored privately. From a clean device (library, friend), change passwords and recovery emails, turn off location sharing, and review app permissions. These are not "secrets"; they are safety.

Every dollar you control and every password you secure increases your options. Options are oxygen.

Breaking Isolation and Finding Support

Abuse thrives in silence. Safety grows in community. Telling **one** person can interrupt the isolation loop.

Choose someone who listens more than they lecture and who will follow your lead. Consider a support group (in person or online with a safe device); hearing "me too" can dissolve shame quickly.(Herman 2015)

At work or school, choose a discreet ally (HR, a supervisor, a counselor). Share only what's necessary and ask for specific accommodations, adjusted hours, escorts, or temporary parking changes. You deserve safety and dignity where you learn and earn.

If faith or family have felt complicated, seek a trauma-informed leader who centers safety, not appearances. The right community will protect you, not pressure you.

Understanding the Brain and Trauma

Long-term abuse trains the brain to scan for danger. "Under stress, the amygdala—the brain's emotional alarm—can become hyperactive, while the prefrontal cortex, responsible for clear thinking and regulation, may go offline. That's why thinking falters during conflict and why sensory cues like sounds, smells, or places can later trigger panic."(Arnsten 2009)

Knowing this biology lifts blame. You're not "weak" for freezing, you're human. Healing is about retraining your nervous system: safe routines, grounding, good sleep when possible, nourishing food, movement, therapy, and compassionate self-talk. The brain is plastic; with repetition, it learns safety again.

Think of it like this: you're teaching your body to believe the good news your mind is trying to send.

Rebuilding Self-Esteem, Courage and Self-Worth

Abuse teaches lies: "You're nothing without me," "No one will believe you," "You're too much/too little." Recovery teaches truth one small action at a time. Start with **winnable** goals: drink water on waking, take a 10-minute walk, make a doctor's appointment, say one boundary aloud. Each small win is a vote for your future self.

Reclaim what got small: your art, your laugh, your friendships, your style. Try "strength spotting" in a notebook—list one strength you used today ("I stayed calm," "I asked for help"). Pair this with **compassionate self-talk**: speak to yourself like you would to someone you love.

Courage isn't the absence of fear; it's movement with fear. Every boundary you set and every act of preparation is courage in motion.

Acronyms for Survival and Healing

Acronyms are more than cute; they're **memory tools** your mind can grab when panic makes thinking hard. (Massen 2019) Here are three examples.

S.A.F.E. — See it; Assess & arrange; Find support; Establish your exit.

When something happens: name it, prep essentials, loop in one trusted person, and keep your plan current.

H.O.P.E. — Hold On, Possibilities Exist.

On hard days, say it out loud. You don't need to see all possibilities to believe they exist.

A.C.T. — Assess risk; Create steps; Take action.

Turn overwhelm into three bullets. Tiny actions compound. Why this works: under stress, the brain prefers simple cues. Acronyms cut through noise and nudge action.

Reflective Exercises, Journal Prompts, and Affirmations

Reflect

- What early signs did I minimize? What will I do next time I see them?

- Which three people/places/media feel safe right now?

- One boundary I'll practice this week is: "__."
  (Write the exact words.)

- What belief did abuse teach me? What is the truer belief I choose now?

Journaling Prompts

- "The first time it happened, my body told me __.
  Next time my body whispers, I will __."

- "A day in my safe life looks like… (hour by hour)."

- "Three strengths I used to survive are __, __, and __. Here's how I'll use them this month."

Affirmations (why they matter):

Abuse can rewire the brain to expect fear and self-blame. Repeating clear, compassionate truths helps build new neural pathways toward safety and worth. Try:

- "What happened wasn't my fault. My healing is my choice."

- "I protect my peace and honor my limits."

- "I am allowed to feel safe, loved, and respected."

- "I am not my worst day. I am my next brave step."

Reconnecting with Joy

Joy after abuse can feel far away. Start small and sensory. Create **Happiness Triggers** you can repeat: a warm-mug ritual with three slow breaths; a 60-second "awe hunt" (find one tiny wonder—sky color, leaf veins, a kind text); a music switch that always softens your shoulders.

Service helps too: send one encouraging message a day. Service heals the server by reminding you that you still have impact. Track your triggers with a one-line log: "Today's spark was __." The point isn't perfection; it's repetition. Repetition rewires.

As your nervous system steadies, joy goes from a surprise to a skill.

Conclusion — Choosing Your Healing

What happened to you was **not your fault**. You didn't cause it, invite it, or deserve it. But here's the power you can claim: you can take ownership of your **healing**. Happiness Triggers aren't cute tricks—they're a daily retraining program for your mind and body, a way to unlearn control and relearn safety, dignity, and joy.

Here's the truth you can stand on: the first time it happens, it's not an accident—no matter what they say. The "I'll never do it again" script is old and dangerous. The data says **three in four** will do it again, often worse. That's why you begin preparing an exit strategy as soon as the line is crossed. Not always to leave tomorrow, but to **choose safety** as soon as you're ready—emotionally, financially, and logistically.

Rebuilding self-esteem and courage takes time, but it's built from small, repeatable acts: a boundary spoken, a password changed, a document saved, a breath taken, a safe person called. Those acts become habits; the habits become identity; the identity becomes freedom. You are not your past. You are your next choice. And you are worthy of a life where peace is normal, love is kind, and joy is yours on purpose.

References

Arnsten, A. F. (2009). Stress signalling pathways that impair prefrontal cortex structure and function. *Nature reviews neuroscience*, 10(6), 410-422. https://doi.org/10.1038/nrn2648

Basile, K. C., Smith, S. G., Kresnow, M., Khatiwada, S., & Leemis, R. W. (2022). The National Intimate Partner and Sexual Violence Survey: 2016/2017 report on sexual violence. *National Center for Injury Prevention and Control, Centers for Disease Control and Prevention.* Accessed online August 13, 2025 at https://stacks.cdc.gov/view/cdc/124625

Centers for Disease Control and Prevention (CDC). (May 16, 2024). About Intimate Partner Violence. *CDC*. Accessed online August 19, 2025 at https://www.cdc.gov/intimate-partner-violence/about/index.html?CDC_AAref_Val=https://www.cdc.gov/violenceprevention/intimatepartnerviolence/prevention/index.html

Esqueda, C. W., & Harrison, L. A. (2005). The influence of gender role stereotypes, the woman's race, and level of provocation and resistance on domestic violence culpability attributions. *Sex Roles*, 53(11), 821-834. https://doi.org/10.1007/11199s-005-8295-1

Grant, T. M., & Cross-Denny, B. (2024). Lethality assessment protocol: Challenges and barriers of implementation for domestic violence victim advocates. *Criminology & Criminal Justice*, 17488958241229928. https://doi.org/10.1177/17488958241229928

Herman, J. L. (2015). *Trauma and recovery: The aftermath of violence--from domestic abuse to political terror.* Hachette UK.

Kearney, M. S., & O'Brien, K. M. (2021). Is it love or is it control? Assessing warning signs of dating violence. *Journal of interpersonal violence*, 36(11-12), 5446-5470. doi: 10.1177/0886260518805105

Kelly, J. B., & Johnson, M. P. (2008). Differentiation among types of intimate partner violence: Research update and implications for interventions. *Family court review*, 46(3), 476-499. https://doi.org/10.1111/j.1744-1617.2008.00215.x

Klein, A. R. (2012). Lethality assessments and the law enforcement response to domestic violence. *Journal of Police Crisis Negotiations*, 12(2), 87-102. https://doi.org/10.1177/0734016817699672

Mulligan, S. (2009). Redefining domestic violence: Using the power and control paradigm for domestic violence legislation. *Children's legal rights journal*, 29, 33.

Murray, C. E., Horton, G. E., Johnson, C. H., Notestine, L., Garr, B., Pow, A. M., ... & Doom, E. (2015). Domestic violence service providers' perceptions of safety planning: A focus group study. *Journal of family violence*, 30(3), 381-392. https://doi.org/10.1007/s10896-015-9674-1

National Domestic Violence Hotline.(ND). *Domestic violence statistics*. Accessed online August 19, 2025 at https://www.thehotline.org/stakeholders/domestic-violence-statistics/

Sabri, B., Tharmarajah, S., Njie-Carr, V. P., Messing, J. T., Loerzel, E., Arscott, J., & Campbell, J. C. (2022). Safety planning with marginalized survivors of intimate partner violence: Challenges of conducting safety planning intervention research with marginalized women. *Trauma, Violence, & Abuse*, 23(5), 1728-1751. https://doi.org/10.1177/15248380211013136

Seelau, S. M., & Seelau, E. P. (2005). Gender-role stereotypes and perceptions of heterosexual, gay and lesbian domestic violence. *Journal of family violence*, 20(6), 363-371. https://doi.org/10.1007/s10896-005-7798-4

Tsopp-Pagan, P. (2024). Silent signs, critical role: why physiotherapists need training on domestic violence–Editorial. *European journal of physiotherapy*, 26(5), 253-255. https://doi.org/10.1080/21679169.2024.2370127

Women, P., Yawn, B., Yawn, R., & Uden, D. (1992). American Medical Association diagnostic and treatment guidelines on domestic violence. *Archives of family medicine*, 1, 39.

World Health Organization. (2021). Violence against women prevalence estimates, 2018. *World Health Organization*. Accessed online August 13, 2025 at https://www.who.int/publications/i/item/9789240022256.

Chapter **16.** Happiness Triggers for Heroes (Veterans & First Responders)

Domestic Embracing the Inner Hero

I grew up in Newark and Brooklyn. The city was always magic to me, and my mom loved it just as much. Every weekend she could, she'd take me on little adventures, Coney Island, the Museum of Natural History, Central Park, Times Square. Those places weren't just outings, they were fuel for my imagination.

My schools were melting pots of culture. In fact, New York City (Queens) is the most diverse city in the world, and to me, diversity wasn't just normal, it was the standard. If a room, party or corporate environment wasn't diverse, something felt off.

Later, when I joined the military, the world got even bigger. I crossed the equator, touched the Arctic Circle, and traveled to places I had only dreamed about: Egypt, Norway, Germany, China, Korea, Japan, Greece, Spain, and Italy. Every stop taught me something new. My childhood and military experiences combined gave me a deep respect and compassion for other cultures, religions, and ways of life. That perspective became one of my greatest strengths.

And you know what? It always reminded me of one of the greatest fictional heroes of all time: Superman, an alien from another galaxy.

As a kid, I devoured Superman comics. He wasn't just my favorite hero because he was strong or could fly. What fascinated me most was that he had powers but had to hide them. That hit close to home for me. Growing up in the hood, being a geek wasn't celebrated. Most of my life I tried to blend in, to cover up the things that made me different. I hid my strengths and capabilities.

But Superman taught me something bigger. That famous "S" on his chest? It doesn't even stand for Superman. On his home planet of Krypton, it's the symbol for hope. And hope is something every one of us needs.

I'm such a fan that I own Superman robes, socks, a coffee mug, even a ring. When friends travel, they bring me Superman gear. Once, someone brought me a Jewish Superman shirt all the way from Israel.

What I also love about Superman is that even heroes wrestle with their dark sides. Remember the movie where he had to face off against the darker version of himself? That's life. We all have shadows we fight. But heroes aren't defined by being perfect, they're defined by showing up anyway. For their country, their communities and their families.

And that's what Happiness Triggers is about: not waiting for the cape, but realizing you already have your own "S", your own hope, inside you.

It's about embracing the hero within, even when life throws you into the dark.

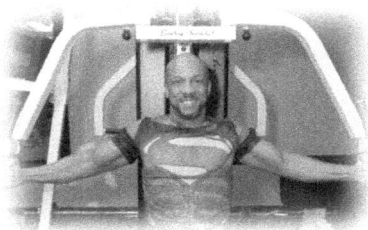

Opening: From Deck to Diagnosis to Destiny

I am a Navy veteran who had the honor of serving on the **USS Boone (FFG-28)** and the **USS Independence**—the oldest aircraft carrier in the Navy at the time. My service took me farther than I ever dreamed: Egypt, Germany, Thailand, China, Greece, Dubai, Korea, Italy, Norway, Spain, across the Arctic Circle, and over the Equator. I crossed the Suez Canal, sailed the Red Sea, and stood in front of the Great Pyramids in awe.

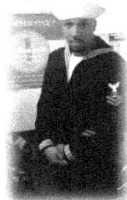

From the outside, it looked like pure adventure. But life at sea was also isolating and unforgiving. We didn't have mental health counselors onboard. No EAP to call from the ship. If you went through something hard, you just kept going because the mission didn't pause for feelings. I didn't realize it then, but this is where my **depression, anxiety, and PTSD** began. The symptoms crept in quietly—restlessness, short fuse, long nights staring at the ceiling—and they stayed.

Today, I am part of the **Hillsborough County Zero Suicide Alliance** and work in public health advocacy to help reduce **veteran homelessness** and build better safety nets for our nation's veterans and first responders.

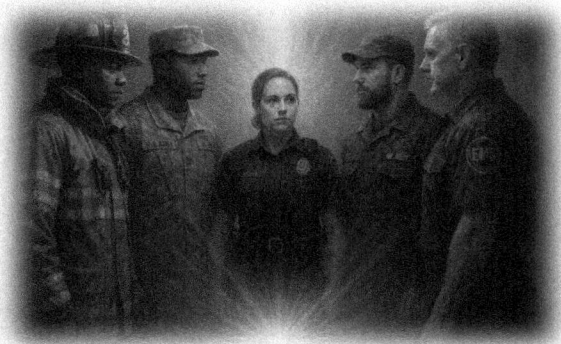

I've seen both sides—serving with pride and, later, struggling to find my footing after service. For a long time, I thought my mental health challenges had me in a chokehold. But I learned something that changed my life: **pain can be transformed into purpose**. What once made me feel powerless is now fuel to help others heal—whether on the battlefield, in the firehouse, inside an ambulance, or at a kitchen table.

This chapter is your rally point. It names the invisible weight you carry, shows where it comes from, and gives you **Happiness Triggers** that don't send you spiraling—but pull you toward healing and joy.

A.N.C.H.O.R. — A Grounding Tool for Heroes

As a Navy veteran, I know the power of an anchor. Out at sea, when storms roll in, the anchor keeps a ship steady and safe from drifting. Life works the same way. When stress, trauma, or strong emotions hit us, we need something simple that keeps us grounded. That's why I created **A.N.C.H.O.R.** — a tool you can use in the heat of the moment to steady yourself, no matter how rough the waters get.

Figure 16.1 illustrates the model described below.

Figure 16.1 A.N.C.H.O.R. Model

A.N.CH.OR.
— A Grounding Tool for Heroes

Attend	Use part of the 5-4-3-2-1 method. Name 2 things you see and 2 things you hear right.
Notice	Notice your body, Are your fists clenched? Is your stomach tight?
Connect	Breathe in slowly through your nose, hold for 3 seconds, then breathe out through your mouth. Do this for at least 90 seconds.
Heartfelt	Say something kind to yourself, like "I've been through worse and made it" or 'Im safe rinow."
Observe	Pick one simple, grounding action; take a sip of water, stretch your arms, or write down a
Reflect	Take 30 seconds to notice what changed; choose the next tiny step.

⚓ **A.N.C.H.O.R. stands for:**

- **A — Attend**: Use part of the *5-4-3-2-1 method*. Name **two things you see** and **two things you hear** right now. This brings you back to the present moment instead of spinning in your head.

- **N — Notice**: Notice your body. Are your fists clenched? Is your stomach tight? Just admitting, *"I feel tense right now,"* helps lower the intensity.

- **C — Connect**: Breathe in slowly through your nose, hold for three seconds, then breathe out through your mouth. Do this for at least **90 seconds**. It creates a pause between your trigger and your response.

- **H — Heartfelt**: Say something kind to yourself, like *"I've been through worse and made it"* or *"I'm safe right now."* Talking to yourself with compassion builds strength instead of shame.

- **O — Observe**: Become an **observer** of your feelings. Imagine you're watching them like clouds passing by. This distance helps you respond with wisdom, not raw emotion.

- **R — Refocus**: Pick one simple, grounding action: take a sip of water, stretch your arms, go for a walk or write down the next step. Small actions shift your brain back into problem-solving mode.

Why This Matters

When life feels overwhelming, your brain's "alarm system" (the amygdala) flips on, pushing you into fight, flight, or freeze. That's survival mode — but it's not always the wisest way to respond. **A.N.C.H.O.R.** gives you a way to pause and take back control. Each step slows your racing mind, calms your body, and creates space between the trigger and your response.

That space is powerful. It's where wisdom lives. It's where you choose a response rooted in strength and calm, instead of being pulled under by old habits, trauma, or raw emotions. Just like an anchor keeps a ship steady in a storm, these steps keep you steady in life's storms — reminding you that you don't have to drift away with every wave that comes your way.

Section 1 — The Weight of Service: Understanding Trauma Exposure

A day you might recognize

Picture a corpsman in the Red Sea responding to a sudden medical emergency—no ER around the corner, only the ship, the ocean, and the responsibility to act. Or a first responder rolling up on a multi-car crash in the rain—lights flashing, people shouting, triage before the ambulance even stops. During the call your training takes over. After the call, your mind keeps playing it back.

What "Trauma" Means (official + plain language)

- **Definition:** Trauma is an emotional response to a terrible event (like a crash, assault, disaster) that has a long-lasting negative impact on behaviors, attitudes, thought processes, etc.(APA, ND) For many in uniform, it's repeated exposure to suffering and danger—not just one event.

- **Plain language:** Your brain's alarm can get stuck "ON." Even when you're safe, your body doesn't always get the message.

Why It Matters

Long-term, unprocessed exposure can lead to PTSD, depression, anxiety, sleep problems, substance misuse, and health issues. It changes how you see yourself and the world.

Signs You Might be Carrying It

- Intrusive memories or nightmares
- Avoiding reminders or routes
- Feeling "on edge," jumpy, or numb
- Trouble sleeping or staying asleep
- Irritability; quick to anger or quick to shut down

Strategies That Actually Help

- **Grounding in 30 seconds:** 5-4-3-2-1 (five things you see; four you touch; three you hear; two you smell; one you taste).

- **Peer decompression:** 10–15 minutes with someone who *gets it* after a hard call or memory.

- **Off-duty ritual:** Change clothes, shower, brief walk, calm playlist—teach your brain "the shift is over."

Quick Reflections

Exercise

Write a few lines about a tough moment you've never processed. What happened? How did you feel then? How do you feel now?

Journaling Prompt

"When I think about the hardest parts of my service/work, I feel ___. One small step I can take this week is ___."

Section 2 — Moral Injury: The Wound to Your Sense of Self

A Moment That Lingers

A firefighter pulls two kids from a burning home. The neighborhood calls him a hero. He can't stop thinking about the third child he could not reach. Or a sailor follows an order, fast and clean... and spends years asking, "Was that right?"

What "Moral Injury" Means (official + plain language)

- **Definition:** Moral injury is the lasting psychological, social, behavioral, and sometimes spiritual impact after an event that violates your moral or ethical code. It's different from fear-based PTSD; it's guilt, shame, or betrayal.(US Department of Veterans Affairs, May 15, 2025)
- **Plain language:** Moral injury feels like a bruise on your conscience. It's the "I should have..." loop. It questions who you are, not just what happened.

Why It Matters

Moral injury can erode identity, trust, and belonging. Left alone, it can fuel isolation, anger, spiritual struggle, depression, or self-harm.

Signs to Watch For

- Persistent guilt, shame, or self-blame

- Withdrawal from people or purpose
- Feeling "contaminated" or unworthy of good things
- Rage at leadership or "the system"
- Spiritual distress; "I can't forgive myself"

A Path to Healing (step by step)

1. **Name the wound:** Write one sentence about the moment and the value it violated.

2. **Name the value beneath it:** Protection? Loyalty? Justice? Compassion?

3. **Restorative action:** Mentor a rookie, volunteer, create art, write a letter, plant a tree, attend a memorial, or support a cause that honors that value.

4. **Talk where you're understood:** Peer groups, chaplain, therapist who **knows moral injury** (ask directly).

5. **Reclaim your story:** You are more than your hardest day.

Quick Reflections

Exercise

"If I could speak to my younger self from that day, I'd say ___."

Journaling Prompt

"The value that was harmed was ___. One way I'll honor it this month is ___."

Section 3 — The Ripple Effect: Secondhand Trauma in Families & Teams

Two Home Scenes (you might know both)

After a tough shift, a police officer comes home quiet. Their partner feels the wall but doesn't know why. The kids tiptoe and test the air like weathercasters: "Is today a storm?"

A paramedic finishes a double and sits at the kitchen table in silence. Their wife wonders if she's done something wrong. The kids stop sharing about school. Nobody names it, but everyone feels it.

What "Secondary Traumatic Stress" Means (official + plain language)

- **Definition:** Secondary traumatic stress is the emotional strain from hearing about another's trauma, often showing PTSD-like symptoms in loved ones and helpers.(Substance Abuse Mental Health Services Administration, February 20, 2025; National Child Traumatic Stress Network, ND)

- **Plain language:** Standing near a fire still burns. Your people can feel your pain even if they weren't at the call.

Why It Matters

If we ignore it, families fracture, kids carry adult worries, partners shut down, and teams lose trust.

Signs in Loved Ones (and coworkers)

- Mood swings; walking on eggshells
- Withdrawing from conversation or family time
- Kids acting "too grown" (becoming caretakers)
- More arguments... or long silences

What Helps at Home (simple things work)

- **Micro-check-ins:** "Today was rough. I'm glad to be home." (You don't have to give details.)
- **Rituals that reconnect:** Weekly pizza night, dog walks, movie on the couch, board games.
- **Age-appropriate windows:** Share small, safe bits so kids know *it isn't their fault.*
- **Family therapy:** A neutral space where everyone gets heard.
- **Personality profile swap:** Each person takes a simple profile, then **presents someone else's results** to the family. One family learned Mom was an introvert; they stopped pushing her into loud plans—and harmony returned.

Quick Reflections

Exercise

List three people most affected by your stress. Write one small way you'll reassure or connect with each this week.

Journaling Prompt

"When I'm quiet or withdrawn, my family might feel ___. One thing I want them to know is ___."

Section 4 — Resilience: Your Invisible Armor

What Resilience Looked Like in My Life

On the **USS Independence**, salt water tried to eat the ship daily. We didn't wait for holes; we **inspected and patched** all the time. That's resilience: steady maintenance. Then life stress-tested my armor.

During the pandemic, **the entertainment industry shut down**, hiring froze, and later strikes followed. I became **unhoused**—not from addiction or being "beyond repair," but because life stacked against me: rising costs, lost income, low housing inventory. When I found a place, **hurricanes** made it unlivable. I was unhoused **again**. Through it all, I still showed up for community meetings, still taught **Mental Health First Aid**, still spoke hope—open about my situation, unashamed. I refused to let anyone judge my whole life by a **snapshot**. Those hard years didn't harden me; they **softened me** into deeper compassion. Our purpose doesn't pause for pain. If I help you while I'm in need—and you help me while you're in need—**all our needs can be met**.

What "Resilience" Means (official + plain language)

- **Definition (APA):** Resilience is the **process and outcome of adapting well** to adversity through mental, emotional, and behavioral flexibility.(APA, ND)
- **Plain language:** It's your bounce-back and bend-without-breaking. It can be trained, like fitness.

Why It Matters

Resilience predicts how you recover and grow. It doesn't erase pain; it lets you live **beyond** it.

Signs of Resilience Growing in You

- You look for solutions, not just problems
- You ask for help without shame
- You stay connected to lifters, not drainers
- You keep a little humor alive—even on hard days

How to Build It (practical)

- **Daily drills**: Stretch, pray/meditate, box-breathing, gratitude (3 small wins a day).

- **Social anchors**: A buddy text chain; a weekly coffee; peer support.

- **Purpose projects**: Mentor a recruit, read to kids at the library, help at a shelter. Service heals the server.

Quick Reflections

Exercise

Write about a time you thought you'd break but didn't. Who helped? What strengths surprised you?

Journaling Prompt

"My resilience is strongest when I ___. One thing I'll do this week to reinforce it is ___."

Section 5 — Happiness Triggers in Action (Rewiring for Joy)

A Small Spark with Big Power

When I was stationed overseas, I had **one song** I played when homesickness hit. For three minutes, my shoulders dropped and my breath slowed. That was my first **Happiness Trigger**—long before I had a name for it.

Reminder: What a "Happiness Trigger" Really Is

- **Definition (our framework):** A Happiness Trigger is an **intentional action or sensory cue** that reliably lifts mood or calms the body.

- **Deeper truth:** It's **not** just a tip or trick. It's a **practice of unlearning** old stress loops and **rewiring** your brain toward joy and regulation. You are teaching your nervous system new defaults—on purpose.

Why It Matters

We've been programmed to react fast and hard. Triggers give you **choice** in the space between stimulus and response. Over time, they **retrain** your brain.

Build Your Kit (acronyms explained with examples)

H.E.R.O. — *How to show up for yourself, fast*

- **H — Humor:** Send a meme to your buddy. Watch a 30-second clip that always gets you. Humor releases pressure so wisdom can speak.

- **E — Engagement:** Text a teammate. Wave to your neighbor. Ask your kid one curious question. Connection counters isolation.

- **R — Reflection:** Pause for 60 seconds. "Name it to tame it." Write two lines in a notebook: *What am I feeling? What do I need?*

- **O — Offer (Kindness):** Hold the door, buy a coffee, encourage a rookie. Service lights a path back to meaning.

S.H.I.E.L.D. — *Your daily protective layers*

- **S — Self-Care:** Hydrate, eat a real meal, sleep hygiene. Your brain can't heal if your body is starving.

- **H — Healthy Choices:** Choose one better option today (walk instead of doom-scroll).

- **I — Intentional Pause:** Stop before reacting. Two deep breaths can save a relationship.

- **E — Express Emotions:** Talk, journal, strum, draw—get it *out*.

- **L — Laughter:** Invite it on purpose. Even a forced smile can flip your state.

- **D — Do Something Meaningful:** 10 minutes on a task that aligns with your values.

B.R.A.V.E. — *A field drill for rough moments*

- **B — Breathe deeply:** In 4, hold 4, out 6 (repeat 4x).

- **R — Reflect on what's good:** One thing going right, no matter how small.

- **A — Acknowledge progress:** "I took one step today."

- **V — Visualize success:** See yourself calm, present, proud.

- **E — Engage community:** Send one text: "Thinking of you." Re-join your unit.

Trigger Ideas You Can Touch and Use

- **Music cue:** A 3-minute track that shifts your mood.

- **Grounding object:** A coin from deployment, a photo in your pocket.

- **Movement burst:** 10 squats, stretch, or a quick walk.

- **Breath drill:** Box breathing (4-4-4-4) or 4-7-8.

- **Sense reset:** Cold water on wrists; peppermint gum; step outside for sunlight.

Practice Plan

- Pick **three triggers** and use them **daily** (not only on bad days).

- Rotate every few weeks so they stay effective.

- Share them with your family and crew so they can help you remember.

Quick Reflections

Exercise

Write five small things that lift you in under one minute. Put the list in your phone's favorites.

Journaling Prompt

"When I feel overwhelmed, I can reach for ____, because it reminds me ____."

Section 6 — Veterans & First Responders: Paths to Belonging and Care

You are **often misunderstood**—even though veterans are a protected group in many settings and first responders are praised in public and left alone in private. Too many veterans are **unhoused**, and too many responders carry their pain off-shift with no place to put it. Sometimes providers haven't lived your life and don't speak your language. It's okay to say, "I need someone who understands military or first responder culture."

Community options that work

- **Veterans' coffee socials** (like in Tampa Bay) and peer groups around the country—your new unit.

- **Skill-to-soul transition:** We trained you to write a résumé. We didn't train you to rebuild **belonging**. Start here: one weekly meetup.

190

- **Healing modalities (pick and mix):**
  - Mind–body: **Yoga, Tai Chi, Mindfulness-Based Stress Reduction**
  - Trauma-focused: **EMDR, EFT/tapping**
  - Creative: **Music, art, dance therapy**
  - Nature/animal: **Equestrian therapy, animal-assisted therapy**
  - Recovery/physio: **Hydrotherapy, light therapy**
  - "Boot-camp" style wellness intensives and retreats

- **Loved ones & secondhand trauma:** Keep using the family tools from Section 3.

Statistics You Requested

- **Veterans (2022): 6,407** suicides; **17.6/day**; about **73–74%** involved firearms (higher share than non-veterans).(US Department of Veterans Affairs, December 2024; Ramchand R & Montoya T. May 22, 2025)

- **Women veterans:** Rates spiked from 2020→2021, then **declined 24.1%** from 2021→2022; firearm share among women veterans also declined in 2022—progress, but vigilance needed.(Miller M, April 1, 2025; DAV 2024)

- **First responders:** Roughly 30% develop behavioral health conditions like PTSD or depression (vs ~20% general population); EMS, fire, law enforcement show elevated suicidal ideation/attempt risk in multiple studies.(Vigil, et al., 2021; SAMHSA, May 2018; Martin, et al., 2017)

Section 7 — Field Guide: Reflections & Exercises (All in One Place)

1. **"Emotional Backpack" (10 minutes)**
   List the three heaviest "rocks" you're carrying. Next to each, write one small **Happiness Trigger** to lighten it.

2. **"Trigger → Reset" Map**
   For each common trigger (sirens, crowds, loneliness), choose a specific reset (breath drill, song, walk, text a buddy).

3. **"Unit Reunion" Letter**
   Write a half-page note to your old unit (military or crew). What do you miss? How can you bring that bond into civilian life now?

4. **"Moral Injury to Meaning"**
   Name the wound → name the value → choose one **restorative action** this month.

5. **Family Personality Exchange (15–30 minutes)**
   Everyone takes a simple profile; each person

presents **another family member's** results. Agree on one small change that respects each person's style.

6. **"3-by-24" Gratitude Drill**
 List three good things from the last 24 hours (tiny counts). Do this for seven days. Notice what shifts.

7. **"Future Me" Visualization (5 minutes)**
Close eyes. Picture your life **one year healed**: where are you, who's there, how do you feel? Write five sentences that start with "I am…"

Conclusion — Your Next Mission Is You (expanded)

You cannot take ownership of what was done to you. It was not your fault. But you *can* take ownership of your healing. That's your mission now.

Happiness Triggers is more than a checklist or a motivational quote. It's a retraining program for your mind and nervous system. It's unlearning old survival wiring and rewiring for joy, calm, connection, and meaning. It starts small—one breath, one song, one text, one walk—and adds up to a different life.

You once served in a unit that had your back. Build that again now—coffee socials, peer circles, family rituals, and honest conversations. Ask for help without shame. Offer help without keeping score. And when you have only a little to give, give that little—because our purpose doesn't pause for pain. If I can help you while I'm still in need, and you can help me while you're still in need, all our needs can be met.

You are not your worst day. You're not a statistic. You are a hero who's still here, still breathing and still becoming. Let the past inform you, not imprison you. Take the next kind step. Then the next.

It wasn't your fault. But it is your healing. And you are absolutely worth the work.

Chapter 16 References

American Psychological Association (APA). (ND). Psychology Topics: Resilience definition. Accessed online August 19, 2025 at https://www.apa.org/topics/resilience

American Psychological Association (APA). (ND). Psychology Topics: Trauma definition. Accessed online August 19, 2025 at https://www.apa.org/topics/trauma

Disabled American Veterans (DAV).(2024). Issue Brief: Women Veterans. DAV. Accessed online August 19, 2025 at chrome-extension://efaidnbmnnnibpcaj-pcglclefindmkaj/https://www.dav.org/wp-content/uploads/Women-Veterans-Issue-Brief-2024.pdf

Martin, C. E., Tran, J. K., & Buser, S. J. (2017). Correlates of suicidality in firefighter/EMS personnel. *Journal of affective disorders*, 208, 177-183. https://doi.org/10.1016/j.jad.2016.08.078

Miller M. (April 1, 2025). Preventing Suicide Among Women Veterans. *VA News*. Accessed online August 19, 2025 at https://news.va.gov/139025/preventing-suicide-among-women-veterans

National Child Traumatic Stress Network.(ND). *Secondary Traumatic Stress*. Accessed online August 19, 2025 at https://www.nctsn.org/trauma-informed-care/secondary-traumatic-stress

Ramchand R & Montoya T.(May 22, 2025). Suicide Among Veterans. *Rand Corporation Research & Commentary*. Accessed online August 19, 2025 at https://www.rand.org/pubs/perspectives/PEA1363-1-v2.html

Substance Abuse Mental Health Services Administration (SAMHSA).(February 20, 2025). Secondary Traumatic

Stress. Accessed online August 19, 2025 at https://www.samhsa.gov/resource/dbhis/secondary-traumatic-stress

Substance Abuse Mental Health Services Administration (SAMHSA).(May 2018). Disaster Technical Assistance Center Supplemental Research Bulletin First Responders: Behavioral Health Concerns, Emergency Response, and Trauma. Accessed online August 16, 2025 at chrome-extension://efaidnbmnnnibpcajpcglclefind-mkaj/https://www.samhsa.gov/sites/default/files/dtac/supplementalresearchbulletin-firstresponders-may2018.pdf

US Department of Veterans Affairs.(May 15, 2025). PTSD: National Center for PTSD. Moral Injury and PTSD. Accessed online August 19, 2025 at https://www.ptsd.va.gov/understand/related/moral_injury_ptsd.asp

US Department of Veterans Affairs.(December 2024). 2024 National Veteran Suicide Prevention ANNUAL REPORT Part 2 of 2: Report Findings. Summary of Key Findings, p. 4. VA Office of Suicide Prevention. Accessed online August 19, 2025 at chrome-extension://efaidnbmnnnibpcajpcglclefind-mkaj/https://www.mentalhealth.va.gov/docs/datasheets/2024/2024-Annual-Report-Part-2-of-2_508.pdf

Vigil, N. H., Beger, S., Gochenour, K. S., Frazier, W. H., Vadeboncoeur, T. F., & Bobrow, B. J. (2021). Suicide Among the Emergency Medical Systems Occupation in the United States. *The western journal of emergency medicine*, 22(2), 326–332.
doi: 10.5811/westjem.2020.10.48742

Chapter 17. Sleep Triggers – Rest as a Pillar of Mental Wellbeing

Sleep is a tricky thing. Sometimes it feels easy to achieve, while other times, it feels like an impossible battle. I've had my share of sleepless nights, even after a long day on set for shows like Law & Order: SVU or Blue Bloods. Despite the physical exhaustion, my mind would stay in "work mode," replaying scenes or running through lines for future shoots. This was especially true during my time portraying Henry Weaver on Gotham— my mind would remain wired for hours after filming, making sleep elusive.

Many of us experience this struggle. After giving everything during the day, you'd think sleep would come easily, but often, our racing minds have a different agenda. Through my experiences, I've learned that sleep isn't just about closing your eyes; it's about calming the mind and preparing the body to rest. As I've grown older, I've realized more and more that sleep is the foundation for everything else. It's the time when our mind and body repair, reset, and recharge.

The Importance of Sleep for Mental Health

Sleep is essential not only for physical recovery but also for mental wellbeing.(Steptoe et al., 2008; Scott et al., 2021) Numerous studies show that poor sleep can exacerbate anxiety, depression, and stress. Without proper rest, our emotional regulation weakens, making it harder to handle everyday challenges.

I've seen firsthand how lack of sleep impacts mental health. During times of high stress—whether juggling multiple projects or managing personal responsibilities—poor sleep would heighten my anxiety. Problems that seemed manageable on a good night's rest felt insurmountable after a few sleepless nights. I've noticed this pattern in my work with the National Association of Mental Illness (NAMI) Hillsborough and a local suicide alliance as well: individuals struggling with mental health crises often face significant sleep disturbances.

Think of your brain like your phone. When the battery is low, your apps run slower, and nothing works as efficiently. Similarly, when you're sleep deprived, the neural pathways that help manage emotions, problem solving, and memory don't function well. That's why prioritizing sleep is essential for mental and emotional resilience.

Creating a Sleep-Inducing Evening Routine

Building a consistent sleep routine isn't just a suggestion—it's a necessity. Sleep hygiene refers to practices that help your body transition from wakefulness to rest. Routines create patterns that train your brain and body to know when it's time to wind down thus aiding in stress management.(Walker, 2017)

Here's a sleep routine that has worked for me and can work for you too:

1. Set a Consistent Sleep Schedule

Go to bed and wake up at the same time every day, even on weekends. This helps regulate your internal clock, making falling asleep easier. I used this method even when my filming schedule was chaotic.

2. Mindfulness Meditation to Calm the Mind

Mindfulness meditation is a great way to calm a racing mind.(KabatZinn, 2003) Whether it's deep breathing, a body scan meditation, or just sitting in silence for 5-10 minutes, mindfulness helps transition your body into a restful state.

When my mind refuses to quiet down after a busy day, I do a guided body scan meditation. I focus on releasing tension in every part of my body, from my toes to my head. This practice helps bring me into the present and calms the mental noise.

3. Record Your Own Affirmations and Guided Meditation

One powerful trick I've discovered is recording my own affirmations or guided meditation in my voice.

Listening to your voice saying things like, "I am safe, I am calm, I deserve rest," can be deeply soothing.

Scientific studies suggest that hearing your own voice creates a sense of familiarity and safety, which helps lower cortisol levels and signals the brain to relax. I've used this technique countless times when other methods failed, and it works because of the personal connection to the voice and the message.

4. Optimize Your Sleep Environment

Your bedroom should be a sanctuary for sleep. During my time working in New York, staying in noisy hotel rooms taught me that environment matters. Simple adjustments—like blackout curtains, a white noise machine, and controlling the room's temperature—make all the difference.

Research shows that the ideal sleep temperature is between 60-67°F. Keeping your room too hot or cold disrupts your body's natural sleep cycle.

5. Limit Screen Time

Blue light from phones, laptops, and TVs disrupts melatonin production, making it harder to fall asleep. As tempting as it is to scroll through social media or check emails before bed, I make it a rule to shut off screens at least an hour before sleeping. Instead, I read or journal to wind down.

6. Sound Therapy and Relaxing Music

Sound therapy, like binaural beats or relaxing music, can trigger a restful state. I've experimented with binaural beats to help shift my brain into a sleep ready state. Calming music has also become one of my favorite ways to wind down after a hectic day.

Managing Insomnia: What to Do When Sleep Won't Come

Insomnia is incredibly frustrating because it often feels like sleep is right there, but just out of reach.(Perlis & Gehrman, 2011) Many clients I've worked with experience insomnia despite their best efforts. The more they tried to sleep, the more anxious they became, which only exacerbated the problem.

Here are a few strategies to manage insomnia:

1. *Don't Stay in Bed Awake:* If you've been in bed for more than 20-30 minutes and can't sleep, get up and do something relaxing like reading. Staying in bed will only make you more anxious.

2. *Avoid Naps:* Although naps might seem like a good idea, they can interfere with nighttime sleep. If you need a nap, keep it short—20 minutes max.

3. *Limit Caffeine and Alcohol:* Both of these can disrupt sleep. Caffeine is a stimulant that stays in your system for hours, and alcohol, though it may help you fall asleep, disrupts deep sleep later in the night.

4. *Consider a Digital Detox:* Too much screen time over stimulates the brain before bed. A client of mine spent two hours a night on social media. Once we replaced that time with a calming routine, her sleep drastically improved.

Letting Go of Control to Achieve Better Sleep

One of the most valuable lessons I've learned about sleep is that sometimes, you have to let go of the need to control it. When I'm too focused on "making" myself sleep, it only creates more anxiety, which in turn keeps me awake. The more I try to force sleep, the further away it feels.

Part of achieving good sleep is surrendering to the process—accepting that sleep might not come instantly and focusing instead on calming your mind. Just as in life, letting go of control is often the key to achieving what you need most.

Reflective Exercise

Find a quiet space where you won't be interrupted. Close your eyes and take five deep breaths, focusing on the sensation of the air entering and leaving your body. Once you feel centered, think about your current life situation and identify one area where stress has been affecting you the most—whether it's work, family, or personal responsibilities.

Visualize yourself in that stressful situation, but this time, imagine using mindfulness or another stress management technique. Picture yourself feeling calm and in control. After this visualization, write down how it felt to handle the stress differently. Reflect on how incorporating this technique into your daily life could help reduce stress and improve your well-being.

Journaling Prompt

Think about a recent situation where you felt overwhelmed by stress or chaos. What were the key factors that contributed to your stress? How did you react to the situation? Now, imagine how you could have approached it differently using stress management techniques like mindfulness, deep breathing, or taking breaks. Write about the specific strategies you could use to better manage stress in the future.

Conclusion — Sleep Is a Cornerstone of Well-being

Sleep isn't just a part of wellbeing—it's a pillar of it. When we neglect sleep, we're neglecting one of the most essential components of our mental and physical health. In a world that never stops, prioritizing rest is more important than ever.

The techniques I've outlined—mindfulness, sound therapy, affirmations, and optimizing your environment—are all tools to help you improve your sleep. Use these tools, be patient with yourself, and remember that sleep is a process of restoration that your mind and body need. When you prioritize sleep, you prioritize every other area of your life.

Chapter 17 References

KabatZinn, J. (2003). Wherever You Go, There You Are: Mindfulness Meditation in Everyday Life. Hachette Books.

Perlis, M. L., & Gehrman, P. R. (2011). Cognitive Behavioral Treatment of Insomnia: A Session-by-Session Guide. Springer.

Scott, A. J., Webb, T. L., Martyn-St James, M., Rowse, G., & Weich, S. (2021). Improving sleep quality leads to better mental health: A meta-analysis of randomised controlled trials. *Sleep medicine reviews*, 60, 101556. https://doi.org/10.1016/j.smrv.2021.101556

Steptoe, A., O'Donnell, K., Marmot, M., & Wardle, J. (2008). Positive affect, psychological well-being, and good sleep. *Journal of psychosomatic research*, 64(4), 409-415. https://doi.org/10.1016/j.jpsychores.2007.11.008

Walker, M. (2017). Why We Sleep: Unlocking the Power of Sleep and Dreams. Scribner.

Chapter 18. Healing the Inner Child – Triggers for Deep Emotional Healing

Many adults believe they're making decisions based on rational experience, but more often than not, it's their inner child driving those decisions. This inner child, shaped by early experiences and emotions, influences how we navigate the world, often without our conscious awareness. Unresolved pain, fear, and unmet emotional needs from childhood can direct much of our behavior as adults, leaving us stuck in patterns that limit our personal growth.

In my work, I've seen countless examples of how unresolved childhood wounds manifest in adulthood—whether it's struggling with confidence, self-worth, relationships, or success. Until we recognize and heal the inner child, we remain trapped in those old, self-limiting patterns.

How the Inner Child Controls Adult Life

The inner child is a psychological part of us that remembers everything from childhood, especially moments of fear, abandonment, or feeling unworthy. (Whitfield,

1987; Weinhold & Weinhold, 2010; Sjöblom et al., 2016; Sjöblom et al., 2021)

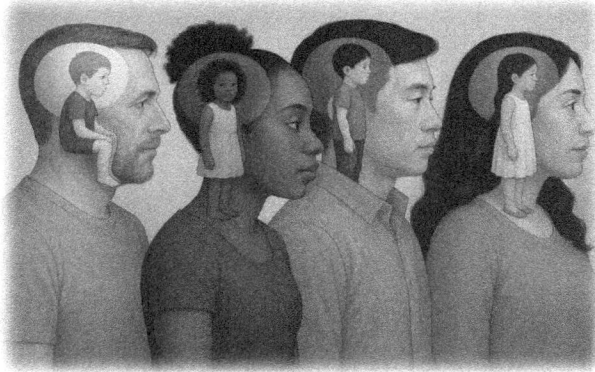

This part of us reacts to situations as though those childhood wounds are still fresh. Even when we think we're in control, our inner child can overreact to perceived rejection, criticism, or abandonment.

Have you ever found yourself reacting disproportionately to a small comment or event? For instance, getting upset when someone cancels plans or feeling deeply hurt by a minor criticism at work. These reactions often stem from old emotional wounds—your inner child is triggered, reacting out of fear, not logic.

Another manifestation is when successful individuals may feel inadequate reflected in their self-esteem despite their life accomplishments or academic performance.(Almousa et al., 2023) They can't shake the feeling that they're never good enough, no matter how much external success they achieve. This is often because the inner child, who may have felt neglected or unworthy in childhood, continues to seek validation.

These unresolved issues, from childhood drive many adults, often without them realizing it. Healing the inner child is necessary for breaking these patterns and regaining control over our lives.

Reparenting Your Inner Child: Taking Back Control

Healing the inner child goes beyond simply acknowledging past trauma. It involves reparenting—becoming the nurturing, loving parent that your inner child needed.(Whitfield, 1987; Wöller et al., 2012) By doing this, you take control as an adult, allowing yourself to make empowered, healthier decisions.

1. Recognize When the Inner Child Is in Control

The first step in healing is to recognize when your inner child is running the show. Are you overreacting in situations where you feel criticized or abandoned? Pause and ask yourself, "Is this my adult self-reacting, or is my inner child acting out of fear?"

I once worked with a client who constantly felt overwhelmed by the need to prove themselves at work. We discovered that this behavior stemmed from their inner child, who was still seeking approval from a critical parent. Recognizing this was the first step in healing.

2. Mindfulness Meditation to Connect with Your Inner Child

Mindfulness can help you reconnect with and understand your inner child.(KabatZinn, 2003) In a quiet space, focus on your breath and visualize yourself as a child. What does this child need? What fears or emotions are they holding onto that need to be released?

I've used mindfulness to reconnect with my inner child, especially during times of stress. By visualizing myself as a child, I can better address feelings of fear or insecurity that surface in my adult life.

3. Affirmations to Rewire Childhood Beliefs

As children, we absorb beliefs from those around us. If we were told we weren't good enough, smart enough, or worthy of love, those beliefs often carry into adulthood. Affirmations help rewrite this narrative.

Affirmations like "I am worthy," "I am enough," or "I am safe" can be powerful tools for healing. Recording these affirmations in your voice makes them even more effective because hearing your own voice creates a sense of trust and familiarity.

Research supports this: hearing affirmations in your voice helps shift negative self-beliefs. I've found that affirmations ease my anxiety and boost my confidence, especially before facing major challenges.

4. The Ladder Method for Overcoming Fears

The Ladder Method helps you confront fears by breaking them into smaller, manageable steps. Instead of diving into a fear head on, you tackle it one rung at a time.

For example, if you fear public speaking because of past ridicule, start by practicing in front of a mirror, then move on to small groups before tackling larger audiences. Gradual exposure helps your inner child feel safe while building your confidence.

I've used the Ladder Method to overcome my fears in stepping into new professional roles. By breaking the fear down into smaller steps, like practicing in front of friends first, I could face bigger challenges with more ease.

5. Play as a Path to Healing

One of the most profound ways to heal your inner child is by allowing yourself to play. As adults, we often lose sight of the joy and creativity that comes from play, but it's essential for emotional healing.

I had a client who reconnected with their playful side by picking up an old hobby—painting. What started as a simple exercise turned into a powerful healing process, allowing them to release emotional baggage they'd been carrying for years.

Releasing the Need for Control

One of the greatest lessons I've learned in healing the inner child is the importance of letting go of control. We often cling tightly to how we think life should go—whether in relationships, careers, or personal goals. When things don't go as planned, we feel frustrated and defeated.

But true healing requires releasing the need to control outcomes. The inner child wants to feel safe, so it clings to control. Teaching this part of yourself to trust and let go is key to finding peace and allowing life to unfold naturally.

I remember trying to force a particular outcome in my career, only to sabotage my own progress. It wasn't until I released control and trusted the process that things started falling into place.

Reflective Exercise

Take 10 minutes to reflect on your current social circle. Make a list of people you regularly interact with, both in person and online. Next to each name, write how they make you feel and whether they contribute positively or negatively to your life. Afterward, consider how you can strengthen the connections that uplift you and set boundaries with those that may drain your energy. As a follow-up, reach out to one person who positively impacts you and express your gratitude for their presence in your life.

Journaling Prompt

Reflect on a time when you felt deeply connected to someone or a group. What emotions did this connection evoke in you? How did it impact your overall mood or outlook on life? If there is someone in your life with whom you wish to deepen your connection, what are some steps you can take to make that happen?

Conclusion — Reclaiming Your Power

Healing the inner child is about reclaiming your power. (Bradshaw, 1990) It's about nurturing and reparenting the childlike part of you that still holds onto old wounds, pain, and insecurities. By doing this, you allow your adult self to step into its full strength, love, and confidence.

The journey to healing your inner child is ongoing, but it's worth it. As you nurture this part of yourself, you'll find more peace, joy, and authenticity in all areas of your life. Connect with your inner child, offer the love and validation they need, and step fully into your power.

Chapter 18 References

Almousa, N. A., Jaloudi, A. N., Abu Suleiman, B. A., Tarawneh, H. M., & Banat, S. M. (2023). Inner Child, Self-Esteem, and Mental Health in Jordanian University Students. *Information Sciences Letters*, 12(9), 2255-2265. http://dx.doi.org/10.18576/isl/120929

Bradshaw, J. (1990). Homecoming: Reclaiming and Championing Your Inner Child. Bantam Books.

Germer, C. K., & Neff, K. D. (2013). The Mindful Self-Compassion Workbook: A Proven Way to Accept Yourself, Build Inner Strength, and Thrive. The Guilford Press.

KabatZinn, J. (2003). Wherever You Go, There You Are: Mindfulness Meditation in Everyday Life. Hachette Books.

Siegel, D. J., & Hartzell, M. (2003). Parenting from the Inside Out: How a Deeper Self-Understanding Can Help You Raise Children Who Thrive. Penguin Group.

Sjöblom, M., Öhrling, K., Prellwitz, M., & Kostenius, C. (2016). Health throughout the lifespan: The phenomenon of the inner child reflected in events during childhood experienced by older persons. *International journal of qualitative studies on health and well-being*, 11(1), 31486. https://doi.org/10.3402/qhw.v11.31486

Sjöblom, M., Jacobsson, L., Öhrling, K., & Kostenius, C. (2021). From 9 to 91: health promotion through the lifecourse—illuminating the inner child. *Health Promotion International*, 36(4), 1062-1071. https://doi.org/10.1093/heapro/daaa132

Whitfield, C. L. (1987). Healing the Child Within: Discovery and Recovery for Adult Children of Dysfunctional Families. Health Communications, Inc.

Weinhold, J. B., & Weinhold, B. K. (2010). Healing Your Aloneness: Finding Love and Wholeness Through Your Inner Child. New World Library.

Wöller, W., Leichsenring, F., Leweke, F., & Kruse, J. (2012). Psychodynamic psychotherapy for posttraumatic stress disorder related to childhood abuse—Principles for a treatment manual. *Bulletin of the Menninger Clinic*, 76(1), 69-93.
https://doi.org/10.1521/bumc.2012.76.1.69

Chapter **19.** The Journey Forward – Cultivating Resilience and Practicing Happiness Triggers

Looking back on my life, it's clear that the journey hasn't been easy or straightforward. From managing talent and producing films to advocating for mental health, my path has been filled with twists, turns, and more than a few stumbles. Whether it was navigating the unpredictable world of boxing with Riddick Bowe or dealing with the chaos of Hollywood, life has thrown its fair share of challenges my way. But here's the thing: it wasn't just ambition or skill that got me through—it was my mindset, resilience, and the Happiness Triggers I learned to rely on.

Spoiler Alert: Reinvention has been a recurring theme in my life. Every setback became a springboard for growth, helping me become stronger and more aligned with my purpose. Whether it was moving from one industry to another or dealing with personal and professional betrayals, I learned that resilience is the secret sauce that helps you not just survive but thrive. And while I didn't always have it all figured out, the one thing I kept coming back to was the importance of mindset and how to shift it.

Resilience: Thriving Through Setbacks

Let's be real—if you've spent time in high pressure industries like boxing or Hollywood, you know resilience isn't just a nice to have trait; it's a survival skill. I've seen deals fall apart, been burned by people I trusted, and been caught in situations where my only choice was to either crumble or rise above. Spoiler alert: I chose to rise.

One of the most memorable lessons in resilience came when I was working as a talent manager. I had a business partner I trusted completely, only to find out that they were making moves behind my back, leaving me in financial limbo. It was one of those gut punch moments where you start questioning everything—your choices, your judgment, and even yourself.

At that point, I had two options: wallow in bitterness or use the setback as a stepping stone. And that's where mindfulness came into play. Instead of reacting in anger, I hit pause. Mindfulness taught me that while I couldn't control what others did, I could control my response. This realization was a game changer. Resilience isn't about avoiding failure—it's about how you bounce back.

Pro tip: When life knocks you down (and trust me, it will), mindfulness gives you the clarity to see the bigger picture. It helps you step outside the chaos and approach challenges with a cool head.

The Mindfulness Approach to Setbacks

Mindfulness isn't just sitting cross legged and chanting "Om" (although that can help, too). It's about being fully present—especially when life throws curveballs. When you're dealing with failure, disappointment, or betrayal, it's easy to get lost in negative thought patterns, replaying the situation over and over. Mindfulness helps you break that cycle.

I had to put mindfulness to the test when I decided to shift gears from talent management and film production to mental health advocacy. The entertainment industry was draining me, and I knew I needed a more meaningful direction. That's when I found my true calling: teaching Teen, Youth, and Adult Mental Health First Aid. It wasn't just a career change—it was a way to find peace and purpose in my work.

But even in this fulfilling new role, mindfulness continued to be my saving grace. I learned to recognize my mental health triggers and knew when to slow down, take a break or step back. The key lesson here is that resilience isn't just about pushing through adversity; it's about knowing when to pause, reflect, and recenter.

The Neuroscience of Resilience and Happiness

Here's where it gets geeky but fun—neuroscience backs up everything I've been talking about. Our brains are like snow covered mountains, and every time we repeat a thought or behavior, we carve a deeper path into the snow. Over time, these paths become well-worn and automatic. But the good news is that we can lay down fresh snow, thanks to a little thing called neuroplasticity.

Mindfulness acts as that fresh layer of snow, allowing you to create new, healthier thought patterns. Studies show that regular mindfulness practice can change the brain's structure, making it easier to manage emotions, focus, and stay calm under pressure. In fact, research published in The Journal of the American Medical Association (JAMA) showed that mindfulness can be just as effective as medication for reducing anxiety.(Hoge, et al., 2023)

Think of your emotions like ocean waves—sometimes choppy, sometimes calm. But deep beneath the surface, there's always stillness. Mindfulness helps you tap into that deeper calm, even when life's waves are crashing around you.

Wrapping Up: Happiness Triggers as Protective Factors

As we conclude this journey of personal growth, resilience, and happiness in the *Second Edition*, I want to emphasize the importance of reframing the way we approach mental health and wellbeing.(Davidson, & McEwen, 2012) We often focus on what's wrong—particularly in the context of trauma, stress, and adversity. One of the most prominent examples is the substantial body of research on Adverse Childhood Experiences (ACEs), which highlights the long-lasting negative effects of early trauma. While this is undoubtedly important, there's an equally significant conversation we need to have about protective factors—the tools, environments, and habits that promote resilience and help shield us from the negative outcomes of adversity.

Adverse Childhood Experiences (ACEs) vs. Protective Factors: A Side-by-Side View

Let's consider Adverse Childhood Experiences (ACEs) for a moment. These are stressful or traumatic events that occur in childhood, such as abuse, neglect, or witnessing domestic violence. Decades of research show that ACEs are linked to higher rates of physical and mental health problems later in life. (Felitti, 2002). From depression and anxiety to chronic illness, ACEs have a well-documented ripple effect.

While understanding the impact of ACEs is vital, we sometimes overlook an essential counterbalance—protective factors. These are the positive influences that mitigate the harmful effects of adversity. Protective factors can include strong social connections, access to mental health resources, the presence of a caring adult, self-regulation skills, and practices that promote psychological resilience—such as the Happiness Triggers we've explored throughout this book.

Let's look at how Happiness Triggers align with protective factors in Table 1 and how they can support
long-term mental health and wellbeing:

Table 19.1. ACEs and Protective Factors

Adverse Childhood Experiences (ACEs)	Protective Factors (Happiness Triggers)
Emotional/Physical Abuse	Practicing mindfulness and meditation to manage stress
Emotional Neglect	Building strong social connections and meaningful relationships
Domestic Violence or Trauma	Engaging in creative expression for emotional release
Parental Separation or Divorce	Developing emotional resilience and using gratitude practices
Household Mental Illness or Substance Abuse	Prioritizing self-care and seeking support systems
Lack of Support or Unstable Environment	Fostering a sense of community and connection

This comparison makes one thing clear: Happiness
Triggers are powerful protective factors. The same way
that ACEs can have a long-lasting negative impact on a
person's life, these triggers can help people cope with
adversity, bounce back from hardships, and cultivate a

sense of purpose and fulfillment. The science behind positive psychology has shown us that we can actively shape our mental health through consistent, small actions. These protective factors become the counterbalance to the negative effects of ACEs, allowing us to thrive despite challenging circumstances.

The Shift: Moving from ACEs to Protective Factors

In many ways, our cultural focus has been to address trauma and adversity—highlighting what goes wrong and its consequences. However, there is growing recognition that we must spend more time building and nurturing protective factors.

Studies have demonstrated that while ACEs are significant predictors of poor outcomes, protective factors can disrupt the pathway from adversity to negative health consequences.(Hughes et al., 2017; Bellis et al., 2017) For example, research shows that individuals who faced trauma but had strong relationships and social support were significantly less likely to experience depression, anxiety, or poor health outcomes. In this way, Happiness Triggers act as a buffer, helping individuals develop emotional resilience even in the face of adversity.

This approach aligns with the positive psychology movement, which suggests that while acknowledging trauma is necessary, we must also invest in practices that foster wellbeing and resilience.(Fredrickson, 2001) From gratitude practices to mindfulness, the tools we've explored throughout this book represent essential protective factors that we can all cultivate, regardless of our backgrounds or past experiences. We have talked about the importance of positive psychology so Figure 19.1 gives a visual reminder of the need to filter out the negative and focus on the positives in life.

Figure 19.1 Filtering Out the Negatives

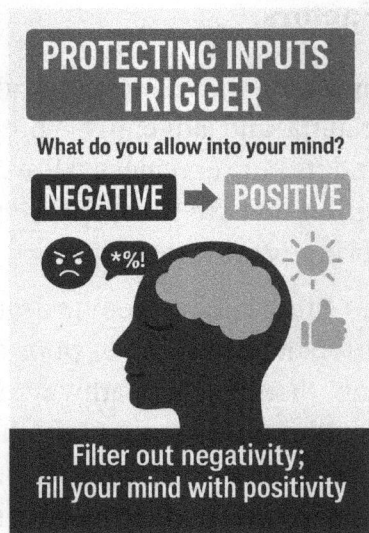

PROTECTING INPUTS
TRIGGER

What do you allow into your mind?

NEGATIVE ➡ POSITIVE

Filter out negativity;
fill your mind with positivity

Building Protective Factors in Daily Life

Now that we've established the importance of Happiness Triggers as protective factors, the next step is to make them part of daily life. Much like brushing your teeth or exercising regularly, incorporating these triggers consistently creates lasting positive change. Protective factors don't just emerge from major life events—

they're built through small, intentional practices repeated over time.

For example:

- **Gratitude** helps shift focus from what's wrong to what's right, building emotional resilience over time.

- **Mindfulness** allows us to stay present, manage stress, and avoid being overwhelmed by negative thoughts.

- **Social connections** provide the support we need to weather life's challenges.

- **Physical exercise and creative expression** reduce stress and boost mood, further protecting us from mental health struggles.

Each of these actions helps create a foundation of psychological safety and resilience—providing us with the mental strength to navigate setbacks and maintain a sense of purpose and happiness.

Bringing It All Together

As you've discovered throughout these pages, happiness is not a destination but a rhythm across all eight dimensions of wellness. Together we explored how to regulate emotions, spark curiosity, nurture your body, strengthen relationships, connect with purpose, find fulfillment at work, build financial resilience, and create supportive environments. Each dimension matters, but it is their harmony that creates lasting happiness. By using the wheel (Figure 1.1 in Chapter 1) as your compass, you've learned how to activate your own triggers for joy, stability, and growth. My hope is that this book has given you not just insight, but practical anchors to keep your life balanced and thriving, no matter what challenges arise.

Conclusion — A Balanced Approach to Wellbeing

While it's essential to address the impact of ACEs and trauma, we need to dedicate just as much energy to building the protective factors that foster growth and resilience. As we've seen throughout this book, *Happiness Triggers*—from gratitude and mindfulness to connection and creative expression—are powerful tools for nurturing mental health and wellbeing. When we actively engage in these practices, we create the conditions for a more fulfilled, joyful life, even in the face of adversity.

The journey forward is about balance: acknowledging the challenges while nurturing the resources that help us thrive. Figure 19.2 provides a final illustration of this point on the choices on which direction we all choose to go.

Figure 19.2 Fork in the Road

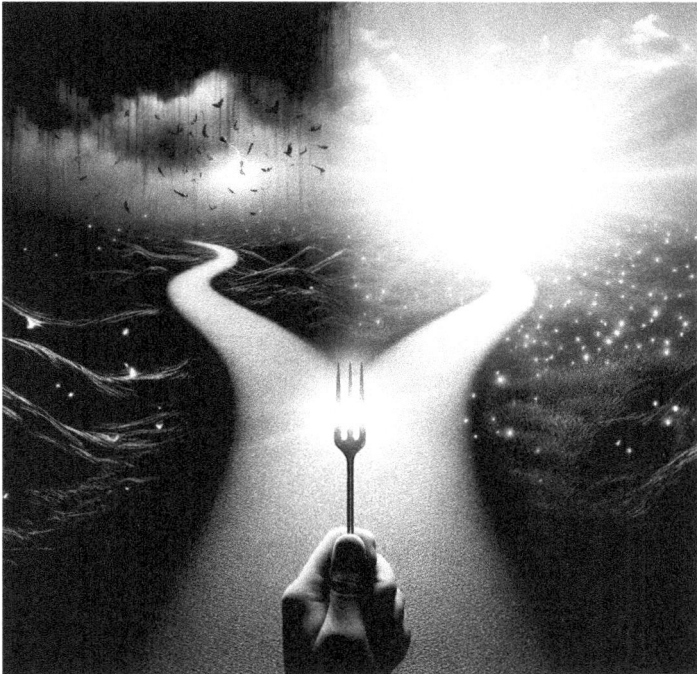

It's important to remember the many points discussed throughout this book when considering the path each of us chooses. By cultivating protective factors daily along with stronger wellness habits and practices, we can foster resilience, happiness, and emotional well-being for the long-term.

Chapter 19 References

Felitti V. J. (2002). The Relation Between Adverse Childhood Experiences and Adult Health: Turning Gold into Lead. *The Permanente Journal*, 6(1), 44–47. https://doi.org/10.7812/TPP/02.994

Bellis, M. A., Hardcastle, K., Ford, K., Hughes, K., Ashton, K., Quigg, Z., & Butler, N. (2017). Does continuous trusted adult support in childhood impart life-course resilience against adverse childhood experiences – a retrospective study on adult health-harming behaviours and mental well-being. *BMC Psychiatry*, 17, 110. https://doi.org/10.1186/s12888-017-1260-z

Davidson, R. J., & McEwen, B. S. (2012). Social influences on neuroplasticity: Stress and interventions to promote well-being. *Nature Neuroscience*, 15(5), 689-695. https://doi.org/10.1038/nn.3093

Fredrickson, B. L. (2001). The role of positive emotions in positive psychology: The broaden-and-build theory of positive emotions. *American Psychologist, 56*(3), 218-226. https://doi.org/10.1037/0003-066X.56.3.218

Hoge EA, Bui E, Mete M, Dutton MA, Baker AW, Simon NM. (2023). Mindfulness-Based Stress Reduction vs Escitalopram for the Treatment of Adults With Anxiety Disorders: A Randomized Clinical Trial. *JAMA Psychiatry*, 80(1):13–21. doi:10.1001/jamapsychiatry.2022.3679

Hughes, K., Bellis, M. A., Hardcastle, K. A., Sethi, D., Butchart, A., Mikton, C., Jones, L., & Dunne, M. P. (2017). The effect of multiple adverse childhood experiences on health: a systematic review and meta-analysis. *The Lancet Public Health*, 2(8), e356–e366.

Epilogue

As I bring this Second Edition of *Happiness Triggers* to a close, I feel both gratitude and excitement. Writing this book has been a journey—one that not only allowed me to explore what makes us thrive but also gave me the privilege of connecting with each of you on this path to fulfillment. My hope is that the pages you've just read serve as a resource, a reminder, and a toolkit you can return to whenever you seek joy, balance, or renewed perspective.

When you look at the cover of *Happiness Triggers*, I hope you feel the invitation it extends. Hands raised with open, colorful palms—each painted with vibrant hues and smiley faces—symbolize the energy of joy, playfulness, and creative expression. The hands represent an openness to life, an embrace of what brings us happiness in its simplest forms, and a reminder that happiness is something we can actively create and share. These elements capture the essence of the book: happiness is within reach, and it can be sparked by everyday moments, unique to each of us.

The act of discovering our Happiness Triggers is an ongoing process. Life will always bring change, challenge, and growth, and the triggers that bring you happiness today may shift tomorrow. That's okay—embrace the evolution, and keep experimenting with the ideas and practices that resonate with you. By remaining open to this journey, you not only empower yourself to live with intention but also inspire those around you to do the same.

I'm thrilled to share that we're taking *Happiness Triggers Second Edition* beyond these pages. Additional insights and information on the book and my work can be found at www.happinesstriggersbook.com. Together, these resources are part of a larger vision to make this journey toward joy accessible, inspiring and personal.

Finally, as we launch this Second Edition into the world, I invite you to stay connected. *Happiness Triggers, Second Edition* was written for you, but the conversation doesn't end here. Let's continue to share, learn, and grow together as a community dedicated to finding happiness in every possible moment.

www.ingramcontent.com/pod-product-compliance
Lightning Source LLC
Chambersburg PA
CBHW032053020426
42335CB00011B/312